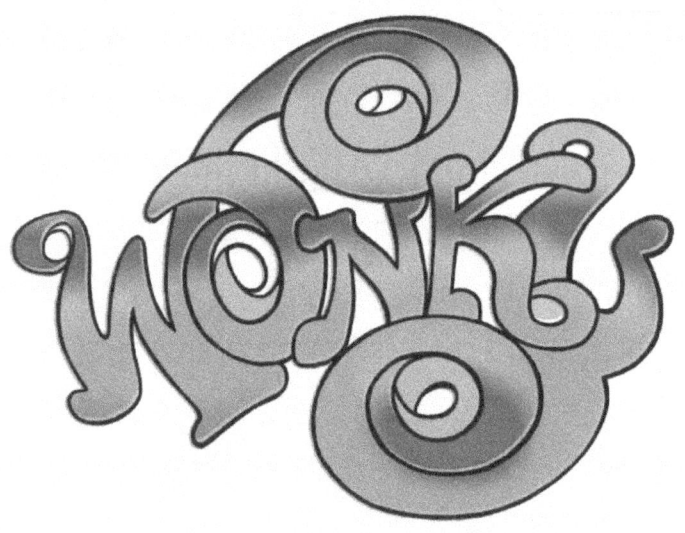

The Guide To Being A Master Edibles Chef

Volume 1:

Cannabis Industry Secrets Revealed

By Jesse Monroe Alexander

Wonky Edibles

Presents

The
Guide To Being A Master
Edibles Chef

Volume 1:

Revealing Cannabis
Industry Secrets

By Jesse Monroe Alexander

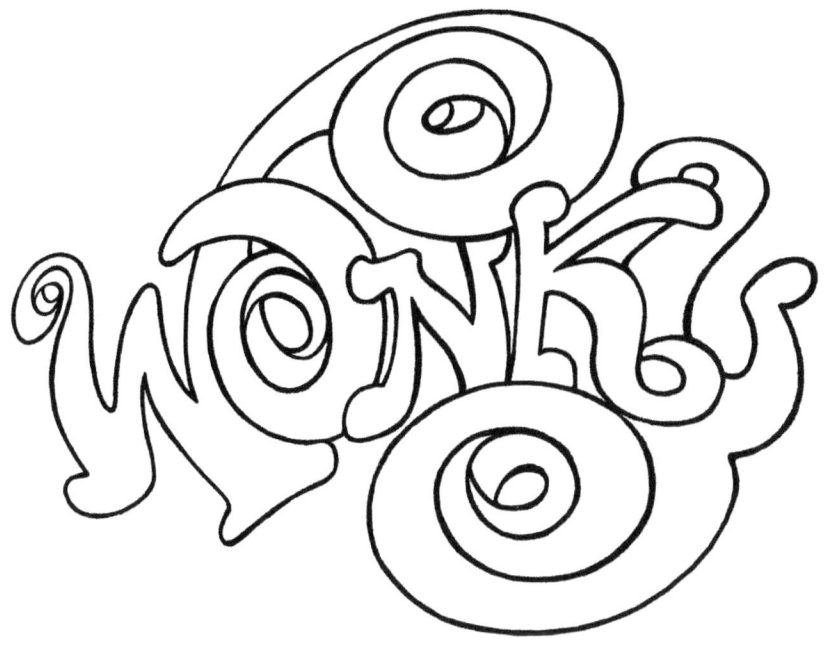

To Naomi, for putting up with not only my shit, but dirty dishes, and anxiety episodes, and for being the best life partner any person could ever ask for.

Also to my family of friends and patients who helped me create amazing medicine and food.

Preface&Disclaimer

As with any book that contains information regarding using illegal substances. Our mission is to inform and entertain the readers and patients. We are in no way liable for any of the readers actions after reading our book. It is not our mission to allow criminals to use our information. The information within is for use by patients and people following legal methods to obtaining their medicine, and for industry activists and workers seeking to expand their knowledge of this amazing medicine.

May your journey with this plant be an enlightening one. I know this rabbit hole is a deep one. We at Wonky hope to expand in volumes as more techniques and information become available.

For now, our information is from facts and available resources as of December 2015 and January 2017. The date when this wild ride begins.

Please be careful to be openminded. As the world of facts suddenly available in the last two decades surrounding these plant species can change your perceptions of family, friends, and even complete strangers.

As laws are changing nationwide regarding cannabis use. Please remember there are millions of prisoners of the war on cannabis that are still unable to say that legalization equated to freedom. These people deserve far more than just being released. They deserve some sort of reparations for the life our laws stripped away from them. To quote Joe Rogan,

"No one deserves to be in jail for a fucking plant."*

*-Quote taken from **The Culture High** directed by Adam Scorgie. Available on Vimeo.

Introduction

"Sticking feathers up your butt, does not make you a chicken." - *Tyler Durdan*

After all these years of growing and making my own medicine. I've come to one clear conclusion.

Not everyone who is a cannabis chef or edible maker, is as skilled as other persons who can infuse cannabis into cuisine.

The days of the green tasting leafy alfalfa infused brownie or cookie, are gone.

The old stories of dumping ditch weed into a crock pot and cooking butter for days. Making your house smell like an amazing mix of wet hay and other strange smells. Are all real stories, we don't deny it, and we can even say some of our close family members have been known to do these exact things in the past.

Other stories of people blowing themselves and others up. Causing damage to homes and apartments, even causing bodily injury. Are becoming too common. People trying to extract the pure medicine using highly flammable and toxic gasses. I know it sounds amazing, but there is news coming out from legal states. Showing that these oils and other concentrates. Can contain trace, and in some cases dangerous large quantities of benzenes and other fossil fuels.

I am going to be the one to say leave this to the licensed professionals in states where this can be done legally and safely. Even then, it should be said that these "fuel" extracts shouldn't be given to sick people. Their bodies are already having a rough time healing. Giving them something that may be harmful isn't in their or your best interest. Patients should stick with organic alcohol or ethanol based extracted concentrates. If trying to obtain the effects of Phoenix Tears or Rick Simpson oil.

***NOTE: If you are unaware of this medical miracle. Please take a moment at your next visit to the internet. Seek out "Run From The Cure" and watch. This information is life changing. Also it is being scientifically proven in several countries labs around the world. ***

We would like to stick with water and dry ice based extractions for the purposes of volume one. Unless otherwise noted in the recipes or ingredients lists. Don't worry, we'll provide a quick guide to doing this yourself. Safely, and with minimal equipment buys. As a patient myself, I understand that any buys could cut into buying your medicine. I will keep it to the bare bones to keep the money in your wallet.

We also want to make sure that all patients do go out and get their referrals if their state has a medical cannabis program. If your not in one of these states. Please consider either moving to a legal state, or becoming an activist for medical cannabis in your state. I know these can be scary ideas. I've done both myself, and even moved to the infamous emerald triangle during a move. A place that will always have a special place in my heart. Both the people, and the plants.

I will cover making some of the easiest edibles, sauces, and the easiest glycerine tincture recipe you'll ever find (something my research has yet to find online. Cover a couple of the biggest edible myths. Also give you some insight into the industry from the fly on the wall perspective.

I will cover much more in depth topics in volume 2. Giving you some insight into planning out harvests to suit your edibles business. If you should spend the money for cannabis training schools. I will also give you the best hoop house for your money to extend your grow season to the maximum. Not to mention recipes the best candies and untapped edibles that will sell out in any market.

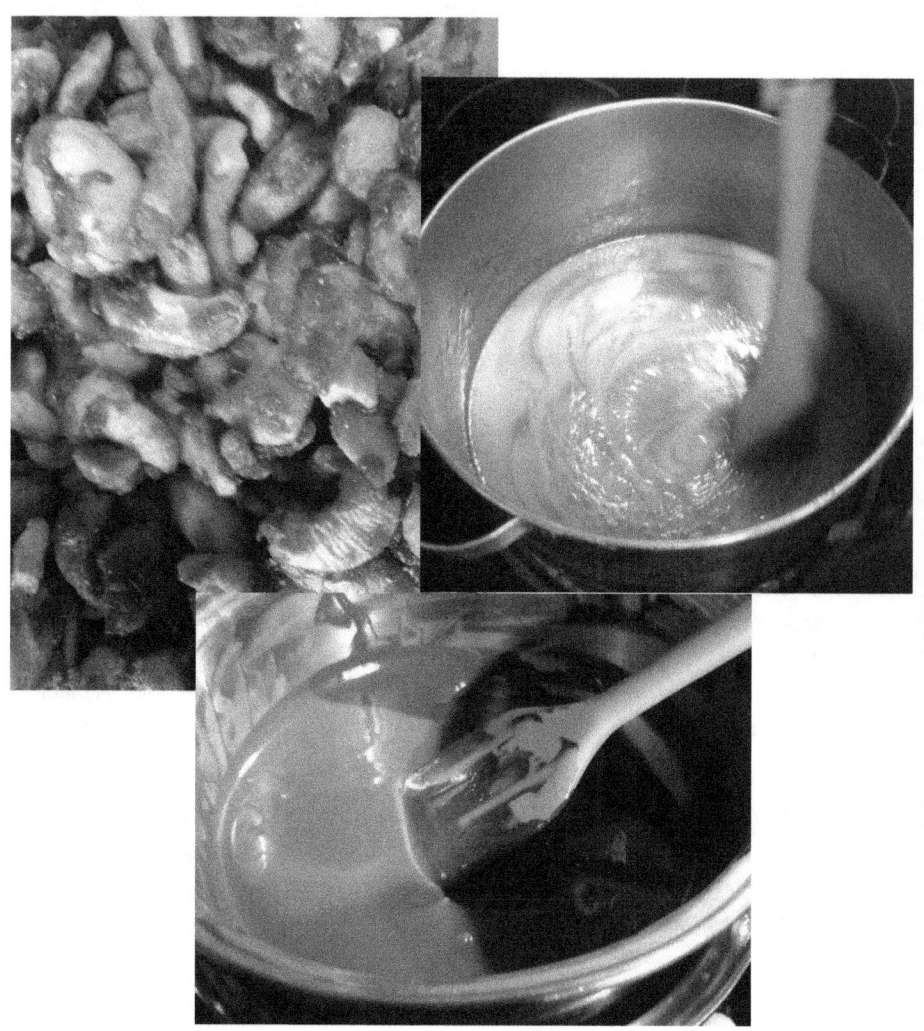

I hope to bring you several more future volumes and even some guides to other aspects of the industry. We both know the industry is growing rapidly, with it will come hacks that can save money, time, and much waste.

Enjoy the book, and we hope that your comments will fuel many more.

One last thing, as you go along wondering how all these secrets can be packed into so few pages. Remember that the easiest explanation is usually the right one. Nothing in this industry should be difficult, and everyone should be able to know the ways we use to create the top products in the world. In fact I feel a bit like Toto, pulling the curtain back on the great and powerful wizard of Oz.

I can't turn you into an instant Jedi edibles master chef, but I will leave you as an apprentice. One that is well on the path to being an edibles Jedi in their own right.

I will leave you with a reading list at the end of the book. To keep increasing your knowledge, and give you the best books from our library. I have a problem buying any cannabis cookbooks or regular books I can find. There are a huge chunk that turned out to be a waste of money. I will make sure you get good information beyond my own meandering ramblings. That way you can spend more money on medicine for edibles.

Why use cannabis?

I would like to start by briefly explaining my own history of cannabis use. As a child, my parents both recreationally used cannabis. My father was many years older than my mother. He grew up in the 1950s, and was considered a hippy during the following decades. I tried it a couple times as a teen, and was not impressed. Like many of my generation the D.A.R.E., I assumed cannabis made you stupid. I had been a small influential child when Ronald Reagan explained that this "dangerous" drug killed brain cells. I am also part of the urinalysis generation, so any drug that stuck around for a month was bad news to me. No one wants to loose their job over a joint on the weekend.

To be completely honest, I was more a stimulant user. Methamphetamine was my drug of choice. An easy drug to become addicted to. Also readily available to small town residents in the western United States. Usually, you hear a wonderful story of an addict going off to rehab. Getting their life together and getting their substance abuse under control. Well, folks, this isn't that story. I moved away from the source of addiction. To arrive in another place where the drug was readily available. It didn't take long, and I was back in the same routine. Only using heavier amounts, and starting to suffer the horrid side effects.

I am not by any means what you'd call stupid. Once I could see that there was a significant chemical dependancy. I began researching the history of addiction and the treatments used. Some seemed barbaric during the late 1800s. I ran across several old stories of laudanum dependency, and opium addicts. Some doctors were treating these patients using cannabis. I understand that methamphetamine is not an opiate. I did see that there may be an underlying process involved. Treat the addiction using a nonaddictive substance, to trick the brain into losing interest in the addiction.

I immediately began to research the truth about cannabis. How the medicines were derived in the old west. Also looking into the plants history reaching back as far into our ancestry as there is a history of us. During this search I found several cases of the same addiction treatment being done in my lifetime up in Vancouver, BC. Not only did it work, the rate of relapse dropped off drastically.

I began to try to saturate my body with as much THC as possible. Eating, smoking, drinking, and even wiping it on my skin. I honestly don't know what strain it was, or the place it came from. It had so many seeds, you only felt ripped off after getting the flowers separated.

After a couple weeks, my body began to lose interest in the stimulant. The heavy THC doses were have a counter effect to the stimulant effects and the withdrawal. Causing my body to sleep, and repair the damage done. I also believe there were compounds that helped repair the neural pathways that were damaged by the drugs. Within weeks, without counseling, or a treatment center. Without even setting foot in a support meeting. I kicked a meth addiction.

This is all completely the opposite of the information provided by law enforcement in my drug abuse resistance education. It didn't match with the drug treatment that I had participated in. It's scheduled by our government as having no known medical uses for gods sake. Yet, I was using it for the treatment of something medical officials spend thousands on with very little positive result.

I continued treatment, which helped my body recover the lost weight, and cleared my skin up. I also found it kept my anxiety, and depression under control. My stresses seemed to lift, and my creativity began to soar. I can say that almost a decade later. I still have no interest in the use of any stimulant. I can thank this amazing plant for giving my life back to me.

OK, take a step back and digest that. That is a true story

I'm not going to let you just take that story and run wild with it. I have no actual numbers to back my statements of others doing this. Most drug treatment offices would call it trading addictions. It's understandable, they make good money treating folks for cannabis addiction. Understand me when I tell you, it worked for me. This needs far more clinical testing. Something the National Institute of Health, and DEA have no interest in at all. I hope to one day see that my story isn't something that rarely happens. It could save thousands of lives, and millions of dollars that currently seem wasted.

I also use the medicine for pain management.

I'm Not A DOCTOR!

Any real thoughts of using cannabis as a medicine, should be discussed with a medical professional that you trust. I have had several doctors visits end in the doctor asking to not discuss cannabis. Most of these doctors also offered large quantities of opiate pain medications instead, but that's another problem altogether.

Many states have services where you can find medical professionals with compassion towards cannabis use. This may not be the case in your state. It is to be hoped that the laws will change soon for you. I live in a state where the dispensaries only recently opened. Although there was legislation regarding it from the beginning over a decade ago. We just now get access to their product. I've had to learn every aspect of this medicine on my own. The state pf Nevada, by law, can't advise marijuana patients on anything except forms.

There are now libraries of information on medical uses of cannabis. If your doctor is unaware of this. Feel free to bring in some literature from the internet and government studies. They recently had to admit THC kills cancer cells. CBD is showing a huge role in epilepsy patients. If the doctor still won't listen. Consider finding new health care.

The Entourage Effect

There are 421 known compounds in cannabis. Several active, and a huge amount of unstudied ones. We are now finding many of the lesser compounds.

Are showing signs of giving us unknown benefits. These groups of compounds do something that the synthetics are not. Marinol, Sativex, and the generics provided by the pharmaceutical companies. Don't contain the lesser compounds, therefore are incapable of providing some of medicinal values of the plant they try to replicate. They may do something for some patients. I am one of the many that it doesn't affect well. Any drug that costs $400 per refill, better do something for the patient. Otherwise they'll save their money, and buy the plant.

The amazing effects of the plant are seen repeatedly. If you want to know if it can help you. Look for the Granny Stormcrow list. A compiled list of medical uses for cannabis. You may be surprised at the multitude of beneficial uses and conditions helped.

Last But Not Least

The world is filled with liars, and cheats. It's filled with bullies, tyrants, and those who would use cannabis as reason to oppress people. I've seen too much of this in my life. I have seen too many people spout lies about a plant they know very little about. I even see courts and parents destroy their next generations lives. I know it seems like keeping what you do with cannabis a secret is the best idea. I offer an alternative. Stop letting them talk this way in your presence. Use the internet to help educate. Almost everyone can pull up facts on the internet and stop propaganda. Write letters to your representatives about changing the law. Stand up for the rights of your peers. Show your support by helping get legislators to change these archaic laws.

To those seeking to profit from the green rush: I'd like to offer a thought on the price of medicines. I stand with a small group of the patients who believe the market needs to drop. The legal market is killing the black market. That doesn't mean it should stay where it is. A considerable drop in valuation would do great things in advancing the end of the war on cannabis and getting sick people access. Drive it to the bottom, and the illegal market will disappear. Ending the war on cannabis.(I will cover this more in a later chapter.)

Just a thought.

Now, let's get to being a master edible chef.

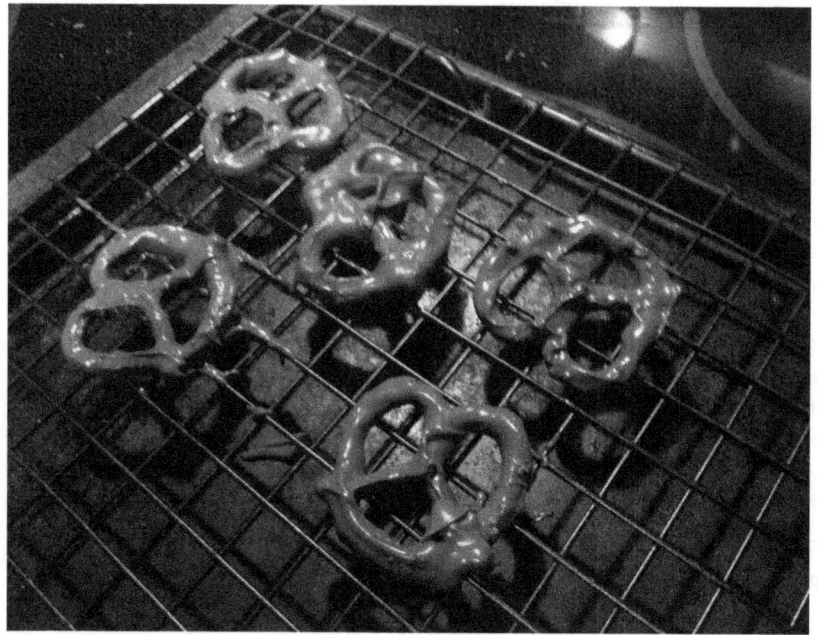

Chapter 2
Basic Tools and Techniques

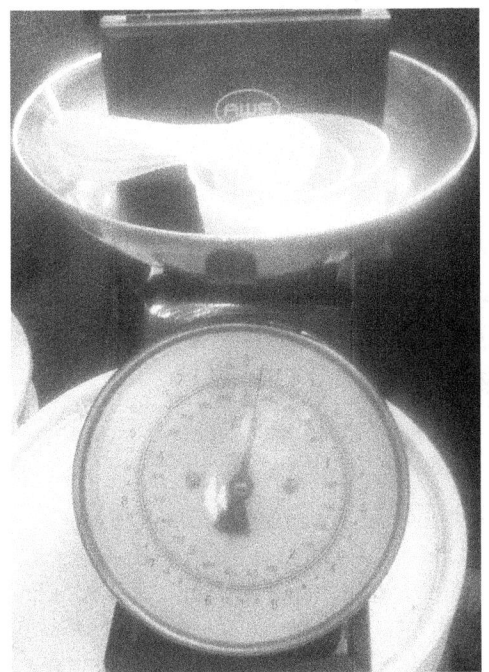

You can begin on whatever budget you want. It can be high end, or bargain hunted. We personally use much of our cooking gear from big box stores and the 99 cent store. Several items may need to be found online to get the best deals. To get the most accurate dosing. Be sure to get the scale that will fit your needs. I've been unlucky a few times and didn't read reviews for products. To end up buying subpar equipment that was unreliable in the long run.

In short, the crappy stuff seemed to break a lot (usually at the most inopportune times).

Extraction Equipment

Hash bags, or Bubble Bags are one of the few necessities. They have many manufacturers and are really a matter of taste and budget. I own some of the more expensive bags. I rarely use many of the screens sticking with a personal preference of three. I also tend to borrow a smaller set of bags and use them more often for dry ice extraction. The larger ones are reserved for rare ice water extractions.

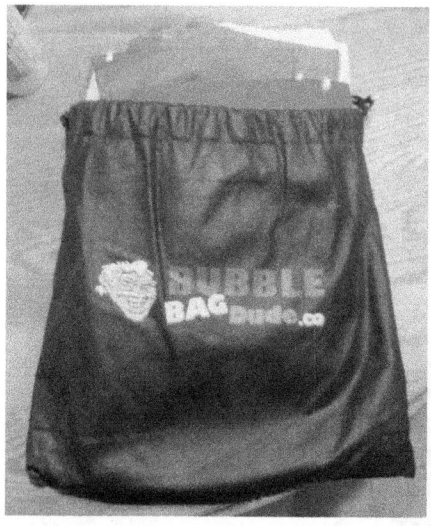

To explain the process simply, the resin glands on the flowers get caught in super fine mesh bags. Concentrating the medicine down to a powder or granule form of hashish.

There is much cool science involved in extraction in the commercial world. If you wander down the baking isle. Check the makeup of the lemon or cherry extracts on the shelves. You should also note that all the extracts are in dark bottles, airtight, and usually an alcohol base. Using this fact and the old cannabis medicine bottles as guide. You should probably use organic alcohol or ethanol if trying to create an outstanding extraction.

Using butane or other fuels may leave many nasty chemicals behind. We also keep advising the reader to leave that kind of fuel extraction to someone with a license and experience. Alcohol boils off at a low temperature, and when done in well ventilated or outdoor areas on an induction heating plate. Provides a safe clean extraction that can do wondrous things to heal the human body. Remember, NO OPEN FLAMES OR SPARKS. ALCOHOL IS HIGHLY FLAMMABLE AS A GAS. IT WILL IGNITE.

We know we can't say enough that this is dangerous. We hope to offer a secondary option for you. A dry ice extraction using a hash bag.

All dry ice extractions can be turned to oil. They also have another CO_2 oil extraction that is being developed in Colorado that looks safe too.

It's more common in the states with legal cannabis.

Compressing the dry ice extraction powder can cause it to become like honey oil. This involves either a rosin press or low temperature setting flat iron, an investment in both money and time. If pondering the purchase, a rosin press runs a few hundred, flat irons run about twenty dollars. I've also simply added a small amount of alcohol to dissolve and let it evaporate off using an automatic rice cooker, metal measuring cup, and electric coffee warmer. This worked well for the low tech version, and cost me under one hundred dollars. A method developed by Rick Simpson, that can easily be scaled down for smaller batches.

In the end, it really comes down to what will work for your needs. Most patients should try to avoid spending more than they have to for readily available tools. Use online retailers like Amazon and eBay. They can provide some tools like milligram scales and micro measuring spoons. These aren't available anywhere local for a decent price. The locally available milligram scale was three times the online price.

Other patients can provide the best source of quality equipment. Most have had to try different stuff. So they may sometimes have sources of tools that online search engines may miss. Also they may have tools that you may prefer that they are looking to offload. I've scored a few cool cooking utensils that way.

Dry Ice Hash Extraction

1. Once you've got the bubble bags. You'll need to find a container that fits snugly inside the bag. Usually you can find 1 or 5 gallon buckets to accommodate the size bag you bought.

2. Fill the container with your dry flowers (you can run trim, but the extraction will be greener and less THC). I fill it halfway, but have seen some others going as far as 2/3 full.

3. Take about a half pound of dry ice for 1 gallon of container. Placing it in the flowers for a few minutes go begin the freezing process. Then stretch the trash (largest micron) bag over the outside of the container. Be careful not to rip the screen material as you lightly stretch the bag.

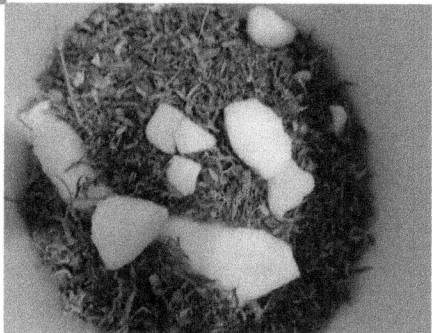

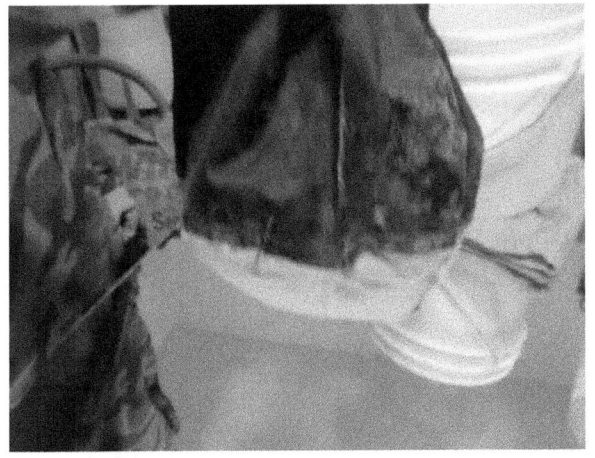

4.Over a large bowl, or large flat clean surface. Shake it vigorously, keeping the container with the screen down. I continue until nothing else comes out of the bag, or it's becoming very leafy green in color. I advise scraping up the extract as the layers of hash as I go. Keeping an eye on the color and amount still extracting. I really enjoy the amount of extraction, without the need of drying and pressing.

5. You can smoke, or infuse this with a carrier instantly with no worry about leftover chemicals for the extraction. That's it. So simple you can do it with no training.

6. Store in an airtight container, and out of direct sunlight to maximize potency.

Be sure to store remaining dry ice properly, or use it to make some cannabis infused root beer. Just make sure that you use it properly and fast. I've never had it last in our home freezer. We open the door too much and it simply evaporates away. DAMN YOU, MUNCHIES!!

A great bonus, this extract retains most turpines. Keeping that original bud smell and flavor profile.

This is something to take advantage of as a master edible chef. Strains like Blueberry, and Cherry Kush can make for spectacular suckers. Chocolope and other earthy strains can make for great chocolates and brownies.

We will cover more of this in the flavor profile chapter. For now you should enjoy your completely safe and clean extract.

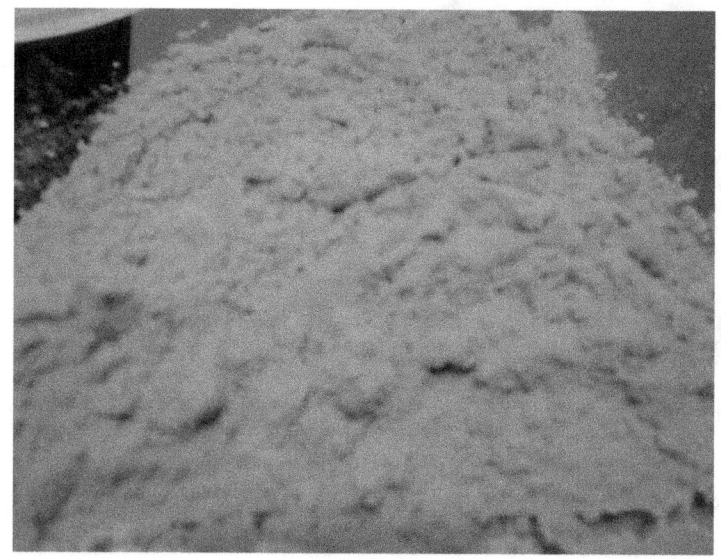

Infusion Process

Add the extract weighed out for correct dosing to carrier(butter, oil, fat of any kind) to small nonreactive saucepan. If you've bought the induction heating source, set temperature to 190 degrees. If using a basic stovetop, insert your candy thermometer to monitor temperature. Maintain temperature for about 30 minutes. I can honestly say that's it. If doing large batches for commercial work you'd use an oven and muffin tins to create pucks for manufacture or sales. That's it, no secret higher held, the time it takes is minimal and lets little plant chlorophyl ruin the flavinoids and terpene profiles in the carrier.

To repeat it, 190 degrees for about 30 minutes. Any longer than 45 and you are extracting green tastes, not improving the high.

Edibles Mythology

I will be dropping these little pages throughout the book. To help answer some of the myths that accompany making edibles. I hope they help with the transition to master edible chef.

First lets tackle the most prominent myth out there.

MYTH #1 - The greener the butter, the stronger the effects.

This is a LIE! Many people cook infused butters or other extractions in crock pots for a day, if not days. This method does carry your extract, just not what you want. After more than an hour or too high of a heat, you begin to break down chlorophyll. This will create the hay like flavor we've almost all had in our edible disappointments.

Effects are based on dosage. The higher the dose, the stronger the effect.

To get the strongest butters, oils, or sublingual carrier. Use the lowest heat setting on your stove. Stir it regularly. Keep it to roughly 30 to 60 minutes. That means 5 minutes over, or under will be just fine.

Make a personal dosing chart to obtain even dosing for your purpose. One gram is 1000 mg of medicine, this is my usual base dose for any patient recipe. It will be weak, and the patient can divide the 1000 mg into the serving amount of any recipe to decipher the actual dosage. You can double the extract if they want until the medicine works

An example: 1 and a half cups of Super Sriracha Cashews contains 1000 mg of extract. One serving is one quarter cup.

6 servings total 166.667mg of extract per serving

This is how to track any dosing. Use it wisely, too much can scare or knock people out. I've even caused hallucinations with a newbie, on accident, I felt bad.

ABOUT AN HOUR, NO MORE. You're wasting time and energy to weaken your own medicine.

Food and Topical Extractions

Now that you have dry ice extract. You can carry that extraction in any fat or oil. When I say any, that means any. Some may not carry well for lab testing. They will however carry the THC and CBD. The most common include coconut oil, olive oil, and butter. These go to carriers can work well for everyone. A few you haven't thought of, may surprise you.

For a nation of stoners and patients. The rarity of quality cannabis infused ice creams and other dairy products is kind of shocking. Yeah, they have it at the clubs and stores. Usually it's not the flavors you find everywhere. To this we offer you the ease of warming the milk or heavy cream or half & half and adding your dry ice extract. The extract, without compression is a sticky powdery crumble, can dissolve easily into most liquids. This opens worlds to most at home chefs. What recipes do you know that require these ingredients. Think outside the box: half & half can become coffee creamer, heavy cream can become whipped cream, milk can become steamed milk for cappuccino. The options now become unlimited.

These tips will help you now that you know the ease of making your own base carriers:

- Milk and other liquids should be only warmed to a simmer. Then monitored and stirred as needed. The dry ice extraction speeds the process of bonding due to it being a resin extract.

- Butters, coconut oil, and olive oil should be stirred and simmered on the lowest stovetop setting for no more than an hour. Any more and it's wasting it.

- If you are using plant material like shake or flower, a jelly press makes for the most return on the carrier oil from the material. **KEEP ALL PLUGS OF USED PLANT MATERIAL IN THE FREEZER. THEY ARE NOT A WASTE YET.**

- Milk, cream, and other liquids should be used quickly. Butter can last longer if stored in a freezer, but still goes bad quickly. Try not to make more than you need to use. Your extract will stay good, and the ingredients will to. Any master edible chef enjoys making up the carriers, it's going to make them a cannabis cup winner.

- If you have any water in the material during coconut oil or olive oil, it can easily make you sick. Make sure to use dry ice extract to ensure no contamination.

- If you want to infuse your olive oil further. Get creative. Garlic, rosemary, and even truffle can be added to increase the flavor profile and value. I imagine chefs nationwide would enjoy a black truffle cannabis oil, I know I would.

- It's always better to make the carrier a little strong. You can always cut it with clean carrier to tame it down. Learn your dosing, and you can dial it in for exact reproduction. Something necessary for most legal states if you plan on forming a legal recognized business.

Topical carriers are not surprisingly, food stuffs. Some of the best bath and body care items are based on food grade ingredients. Cocoa butter, shea butter, almond oil, sunflower oil, and if you check any of the high end labels you'll get the picture. I've made lotion bars, salves, and even a version of an Asian burning cream for sore muscles (I'm gonna give you that one a little later in the book series). So as they are the same ingredients. They are just as simple to make cannabis infused versions.

The ingredients that get turned into carriers, become the stars in your dish or bath and body product. Treat them as such, and use the best you can get.

Basic Dosing

This chart on the following page will give you a basic idea of your dosing. This is a per serving dose. So let me explain by example. You want to make cannabutter for a cookie recipe. You infuse a cup of melted butter with 14 tsp (7 grams) of dry ice extract. The finished cookie recipe says it makes 36 cookies. The 7 grams, or 7000 milligrams, divides out to 194.44mg per each of the 36 cookies.

Gram/mg	Teaspoon
.5 gram/ 500mg	1 tsp.
1 gram/ 1000mg	2 tsp.
Example: 7.5 grams/7500mg	15 tsp.

To increase the dosage of each cookies simply make the recipe into 24 cookies and have each be 291.67mg.

This doesn't change. You divide the total amount of extract, by the servings of the recipe. That's right, if the recipe says how many servings. You can plan out the exact dose per serving. An example, a dinner recipe says 6 servings. You can then add the appropriate milligrams: 12 teaspoons for 1000 mg per serving, 6 teaspoons for a 500 mg, and so on.

Once you get the hang of deciphering your own edibles dosage. It makes the whole edibles market far less scary. You'll know the effects of your 250 mg edible, so you can expect the same from an equivalent edible.

This also makes it so you can break certain edibles dosages, like nuts, to the exact milligram per nut. Good for many child and epilepsy patients, this same breakdown works for CBD dosages. Making the option available for CBD candies and chocolates.

The only thing I'm going to say about recommended dosages. Is to offer my own experience. I am a high tolerance patient, which means that the clubs don't sell many edibles strong enough for me. My base edible dose is in the 250 mg range. If I am in pain, it can go far higher. I can eat upwards of 1500-3000mg. This would floor most people that aren't use to edibles. I have many years of building up a tolerance to the effects. This isn't something to brag about, it's simply my reality as a patient.

Everyone has different needs, and will have different doses. I will venture to say that there will be a handful of people who will not be pleased by dispensary dosages, and may never be. This is just one of those things. I advise any entrepreneur to make a few super powerful items to try to keep these patients happy. Just remember that most people aren't like that. I would hope that most new companies would start at 500 mg per edible pack. That will be worth the price for most people, and still not too powerful for newbies.

If you want more information on dosing. I can highly recommend "The Ganja Kitchen Revolution" by Jessica Catalano available through Green Candy Press. She has written one of the finest cannabis cookbooks, with the BEST dosing information I've ever read. My hat is off to her, and the work she did to make that book. Please go out and get it. This book should be on your shelf. Her recipes for basic ingredients are awesome.

Speaking of ingredients, lets move on.

Ingredients Make You, Or Break You.

I've been lucky enough to be an organic farmer for the past 4 years. One thing I'm proud of are the ingredients I use. I know that many edibles companies want people to think that this is difficult. Most people are using box mixes or recipes

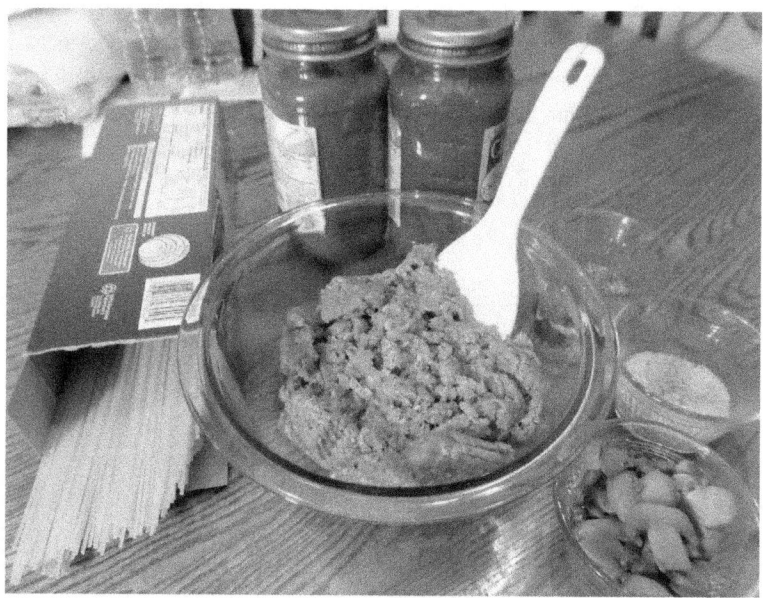

crafted by chefs trying to enhance the existing flavors within. Barely any normal recipes are crafted to handle the flavors of cannabis. Only the edibles chefs dare to tread into the unknown and craft special recipes of amazing ingredients that enhance the cannabis flavor profile.

It's a lot like adding an extra ingredient to any other recipe. You may need to experiment to find the right strain for the right recipe. Obtaining the best flavor matches you can find.

Flavor Profiles

Most strains today have a review page online. Describing flavors and even naming some after their intense aromas. I've taken to being a connoisseur, describing it like most wine enthusiasts. To help you learn this technique. Lets give you a quick rundown on how to determine the flavors of your medicine.

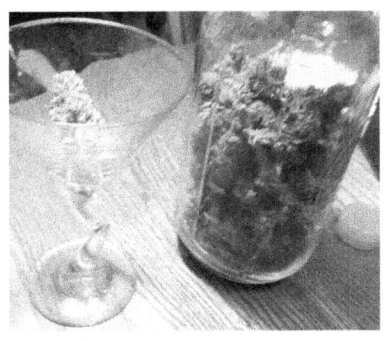

1.Grab a clean glass or jar.

2.Take a bud and break it down (or a small amount of dry ice extract) and pour the ground material into the glass.

3.Most turpenes are quickly released and dissipated. So stick your nose into the glass and close your eyes. Take a deep slow breath through your nose. Then describe the flavors you sense. Move the material around and do it again. As the smell dissipates, your descriptions give you an idea of where to begin.

4. Take the material and smoke it. Do the same technique for the flavor description of the smoke or vapor. Note the effects for the possible later time to eat it. Sativas tend to not make people sleepy, Indica's the knock you out kind(remember in-da-couch). This can sometimes be used for designing breakfast and lunchtime treats for heavy use patients.

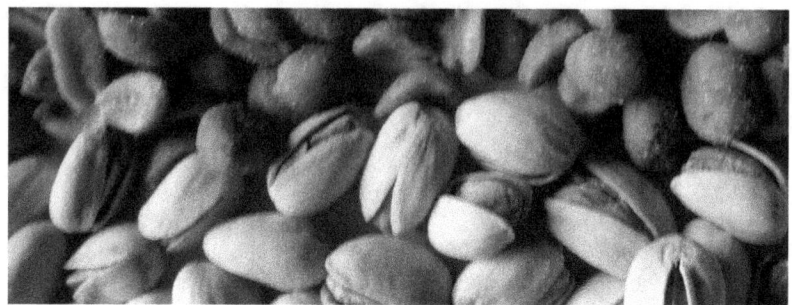

This is where masters really begin. If it had a citrus smell, or mango can I use that? Did it have a cheese smell? What would that smell improve upon? Is it too powerful smelling to miss? Was there a peppery taste?

So we start the search to match this strain with a recipe you love to eat. If your going to make an edible. Make something that you truly love to eat. You'll find yourself more willing to experiment on foods you like eating. Most people who make recipes from scratch can attest to doing this anyway, it's time to get used to it.

Please make sure to use good ingredients regardless of the recipe. Good doesn't mean expensive. It means avoiding foods that may be questionable, over processed or full of preservatives. Crappy chocolate will taste like crappy chocolate regardless of cannabis. If it tastes good before, it will usually taste good after. We obtain good ingredients from our local food co-op and can even order in bulk if necessary. It also gives us access to our local farmers. Which means amazing eggs, honey, ginger, and so much more.

If you're going to be a master, it's time to think of this as a competition, friendly, but still a competition. If you watch any competition cooking show, you're going to hear the judges tear the dishes apart. It's time to be that discerning concerning your edibles. I will tell people exactly what I think of their edibles. I also ask that people tell me what they really think, and how strong the cannabis taste is.

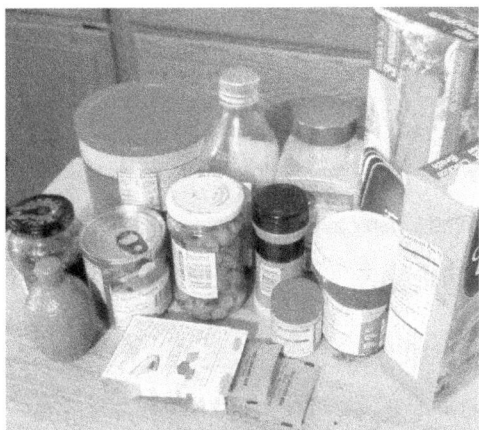 My food is that important, and so should yours be.

I also like the ever expanding foodie world, these amazing chefs and restaurants can provide great insight into making the best edibles in the world. One chef inspired dish can even provide you the inspiration for a possible Cannabis Cup winner. The ideas can come from anywhere.

I like to take my favorite foods and make them healthier, all while tainting them to a powerful medicine that tastes great. This should be your goal in this endeavor, at least if you really want to be the best.

Compounding Ingredients

Let's start this with a story. Back during my first year as a patient, I was unaware of compounding ingredients. I was happily making brownies, and chocolate chip cookies, and even made some Mac and cheese. All this stuff was good, and from the same batch of butter. One night I decided that some peanut butter cookies sounded good. Being the edibles chef I am, I made myself some and gave the rest away to other patients in my family. These people had enjoyed my other recipes, but found these cookies were far stronger. I tried them and found the effect to be multiplied by at least 2 if not 3.

Edibles Mythology

Myth #2 - An edible will be the same, regardless of when you take it.

FALSE
There are subtle things that can effect the strength of an edible. Some of which you may not have taken into account.

These two factors need to be kept in mind when eating an edible.

What was the time of your last meal?

What was that last meal made up of?

These two questions can help prevent wasting medicine. If you've ever eaten a big meal. You'll understand what I mean by food bogging your system down. With too much food in your stomach. You may find that taking an edible will seem useless. Your body will actually take up the THC and be too busy to process it with the other foods being consumed already.

Wait...

Simply waiting a half hour to an hour will allow your body to finish working on your meal. If it's a thanksgiving size meal, you may want to start the meal with the edible, wait for it to kick in, and then go after the food.

This may not work in all cases. My experiments with infused spaghetti sauce seem to only work well if I stop eating it after a small plate. The more pasta and sauce and bread, the less the effects.

NOTE: I am not a scientist, nor an expert. These are my own conclusions, but this does make complete dietary sense. So draw what you will.

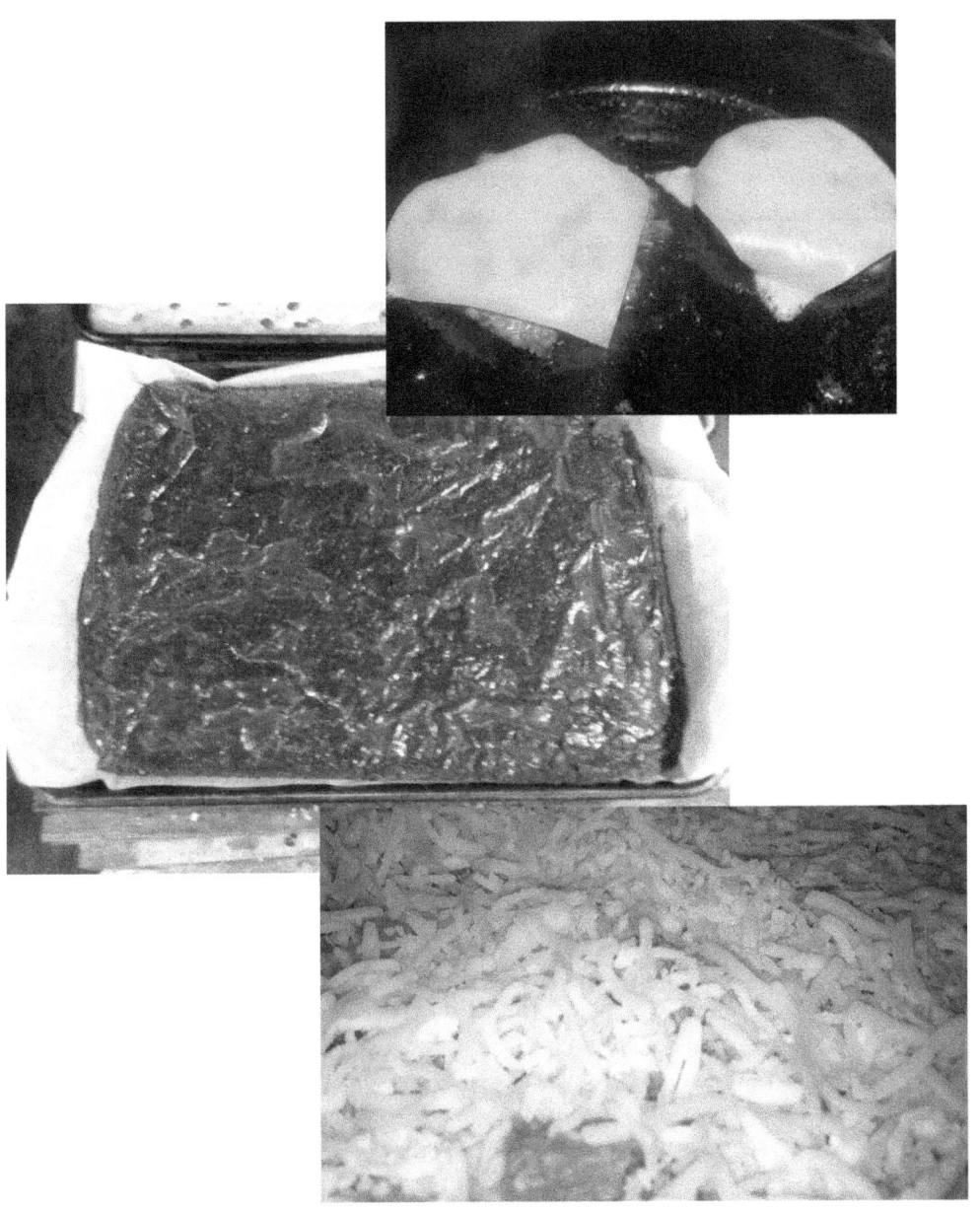

How could that be? I had made these all from the same butter. Exactly the same strength, but these were more potent? Was I missing something?

The answer lies in the compounding effect of certain other ingredients. Unbeknownst to me then, all natural peanut butter, can increase THC potency inside the human body. This was amazing to me, and still is as I find other foods that increase the potency of my medicine.

Ingredients that can compound the effects include:

- All natural peanut butter   - Caffeine

- Coffee   - Mango puree or juice

- Alcohol   - natural peanut oil

These can bring a powerful punch to edibles that may only contain a low dosage. Be careful to not overdose when using compound effects. Try to use more sativa to keep patients from falling asleep. Indica strains and compound ingredients tends to make most people very groggy. This is also one of the ways that can cause some people to hallucinate on the high amounts of active ingredients.

Recipes

The bulk of this book is going to be these recipes. Volume one is going to get you started in the right direction. I decided to give you a few recipes in each area. These will give you the tools to expand and take your own edible journey, into the wild and beyond.

I picked a few things that will give you the necessary skills to compete with the industry, or at least land you a job as an edibles maker or assistant to. Before we get started I wanted to say a few things about creating food.

This craft, is a way of expressing love without words. Food is love, and edibles should be thought of doubly so. We are creating the finest medicinal food, with the best ingredients and extracts. If you think about it, you should be enthralled at the opportunity before you. To be able to make someone feel longing for a food that will have an impact on and imprint upon this person forever.

Are you happy with just making food people will be OK with? Just OK...

I, for one, hope you would show any person that eats your edibles. That this can be a culinary art form that can rival some of the best three star chefs on their best days.

As we move forward you'll notice the dessert section to be a bit more tips and tricks with easy recipes that can scale up to even that largest edible makers needs. I hope by that point you'll have gotten the point I keep trying to hammer in. Any recipe can be infused with cannabis. It's your job to make it awesome.

Have fun with these great recipes!

Breakfast

Magic Morning Oatmeal

Breakfast Burrito

Daykiller Coffee Cake

Morning Drink mixes

Uncle Guy's Humboldt County Mocha Mix

Lunch & Dinner

Cheeseburger

Meatloaf

Meatball Sub

Flatbread or Pizza

Desserts

Homemade Marshmallows

Making Chocolate

Making Cookies

Making Ice Cream

Making Cakes and Breads

Snacks

Sweet Sriracha Cashews

Grammie Annes Candied Nuts

Beef Jerky

Dehydrated Fruit Purees

Popcorn Recipes

Sauces

Heavenly Hot Sauce

Badass BBQ Sauce

Emerald Triangle Ranch Dressing

Chillin' Chocolate Sauce

Breakfast

Magic Morning Oatmeal

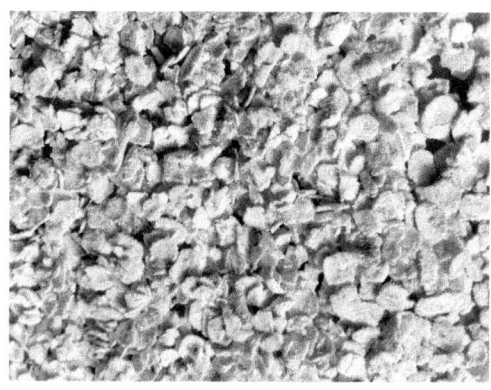

Quick Oats

Boiling water

Plain Yogurt

1/8 cup cannabis infused milk per serving

Raisins, dried blueberries, or other dried fruit

Brown sugar or honey to taste

Bring all dry ingredients and infused milk together in a bowl. Add boiling water to desired consistency. Add a dollop of your favorite yogurt, sprinkle with the brown sugar or honey.

As this recipe is scaleable to accommodate even the largest family gathering breakfast. I make it into a dry bulk mix and then add wet ingredients. Giving this treat with a huge breakfast will bring down the level of the effects. I tend to medicate with this and an infused cup of coffee.

Breakfast Burritos

6 eggs scrambled and slightly underdone

8 tortillas

1 c shredded pepper jack cheese

2 c cooked hash browns

Chorizo or breakfast sausage, browned and drained

1/2 c sour cream(optional)

1/2 c chopped lettuce

1/2 c salsa

8 doses of cannabis extract - separated out

Preheat oven to 325 degrees for immediate cooking.

Add eggs to warmed tortillas, and sprinkle dry ice cannabis extract over evenly. Add cheese and remaining ingredients evenly. Wrap and place into preheated oven for about 15 minutes or until eggs and cheese are fully cooked. Breakfast burritos can be easily pre-made and then frozen for quick access. Combine ingredients to your liking I like to dip in sour cream.

To freeze: Wrap burritos in parchment paper and aluminum foil. Best if eaten within a month.

Warning: Increasing the size of the burritos will only hamper the uptake of THC. Keep them to a medium size for a better high.

Daykiller Coffee Cake

2 1/2 c AP Flour

1 1/2 c packed brown sugar

1/2 t salt

2/3 c butter

2 t baking powder

1/2 t ground cinnamon

1/2 t ground nutmeg

2 eggs, beaten

1 1/3 c buttermilk (or add 1 T lemon juice to regular milk, stir, let stand 5 min).

1/2 c chopped nuts, optional

2 1/2 grams dry ice extract

Grease 13x9 pan and set aside. Combine flour, extract, brown sugar, and salt. Cut in butter until mixture resembles crumbs and set aside 1/2 c of mixture. Stir in remaining dry ingredients to mixture.

Combine eggs and buttermilk and add all ingredients at once to dry, mixing well. Spoon batter into prepared pan, and sprinkle with remaining crumb mixture and nuts. Bake at 350 for 35-40 minutes or till a toothpick comes out clean.

Serve warm or cool and vacuum seal for later consumption.

Additional variations on coffee cakes:

Fruit Buckle Up

- Add 2 c fruit of choice after spooning the batter into the pan. Our recommendation is blackberry, or raspberry. Any frozen or fresh cut fruit will do.

Coffee Cake Pops

- Cutting plain coffee cake into 1x1 squares. Compress the cake squares into a ball using disposable gloves. Add 1/2 t instant coffee to 1 cup chocolate melting nibs in double boiler (you can double infuse by adding more extract to the chocolate mixture). Using candy sticks inserted into the cake ball, dip halfway into melted chocolate mixture. Set to cool it should make about 100 pops at about 25 mg. If you want more chocolate, make another batch or double it if your boiler is large enough.

Muffins

- Easy, use a muffin tin, divide the number of evenly scooped muffins into 2500 to determine your dosages.

- Also the same for small loaf pans.

Warning: Do not attempt much if you ingest large amounts of this coffee cake. We call it Daykiller for a reason. The cake pops make it easier as the dosage is far lower than the original recipe. Eat at your own risk.

Morning Drink Mixes

All hot drinks could be infused. They can also be served over ice for a delightful summer treat. The trick is to add a small amount of cream or milk to bond with the dry ice extract. Even adding it to packets of drinks from the store this makes this a true trick of the trade.

The bonus trick is now you have something to use up all the excess tubes your pre-rolls come in, and you can mix large amounts into the bulk reusable dispensary packaging. Adding the extract directly to any hot cocoa, cappuccino, or chai mix in a tube creates a single serving treat that doesn't smell like cannabis, and cannot be considered consumable until mixed with hot water which makes active the milk solids. Making it safe for transportation for all the patients who need to travel.

This will save you lots if you enjoy the new infused Keurig cups, or have enjoyed a cannabis drink from a recreational state.

Chai Delight

Chai is an easy cover for any residual taste of cannabis, think of it as our cultures version of Bhang when you add dry ice extract. Chai mix, organic and far easier than mixing your own, is really the best way to make this with consistency. If you do enjoying making your own there are amazing recipes online. Here is ours starting with the base and then spices:

1 c nonfat dry milk powder
1 c powdered nondairy creamer
1 c French vanilla flavored powdered nondairy creamer
2 1/2 c white sugar
1 1/2 c unsweetened instant tea

2 teaspoons ground ginger
2 teaspoons ground cinnamon

1 t ground cloves
1 t ground cardamom

3.5 g of dry ice extract

Combine milk powder, nondairy creamer, vanilla flavored creamer, sugar and instant tea in a bowl. Stir in ginger, cinnamon, cloves and cardamom. Pour mixture 1 cup at a time into a food processor and blend until a fine powder. Add heaping 2 T to a coffee cup of hot water. (optional spices 1 t nutmeg and allspice, 1/4 t white pepper). Dosing should be about 100 mg per cup, but the heaping changes the exact amount per cup.

Spiced and Regular Hot Cocoa

Spiced cocoa, slightly changed from the original Mayan and Aztec treat, was actually probably meant to find a home as an infused cannabis drink. Hot cocoa mix can be elevated using cinnamon, nutmeg, and cayenne to enhance all the flavors. Using the more spicy flavored cannabis strains can also enhance these flavors further. Growing your own cayenne peppers to try also gives your blend it's own unique flavor profile.

For the purist here's a full recipe of both regular and spiced:

Regular Hot Cocoa Mix

3 1/2 c nonfat dry milk powder

2 c sifted powdered sugar

1 c powdered nondairy creamer

1/2 c unsweetened cocoa powder

1.6 g dry ice extract

Using sifter mix well into a medium bowl. Store in an airtight container. Makes 16 servings at 1/3 c mix to 3/4 c boiling water. Making each dose about 100 mg of extract.

Spiced Hot Cocoa Mix

3 1/2 c nonfat dry milk powder

2 c sifted powdered sugar

1 c powdered nondairy creamer

1/2 c unsweetened cocoa powder

1 t ground cinnamon

1/2 t ground cayenne pepper

1/2 t ground nutmeg

1.6 g dry ice extract

Using sifter mix well into a medium bowl. Store in an airtight container. Makes 16 servings at 1/3 c mix to 3/4 c boiling water. Making each dose about 100 mg of extract.

Uncle Guy's Humboldt County Mocha Mix

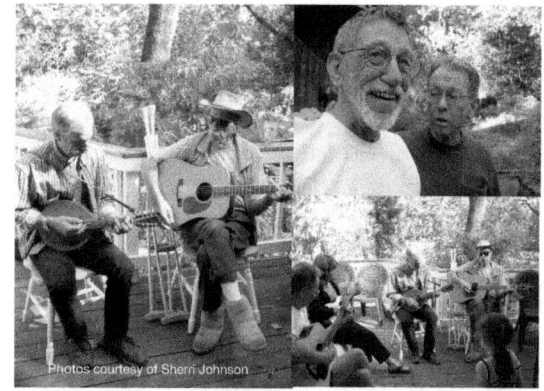

3 1/2 c nonfat dry milk powder

2 c sifted powdered sugar

1 c powdered nondairy creamer

1/2 c unsweetened cocoa powder

1/2 c instant coffee crystals

1.6 g dry ice extract

Photos courtesy of Sherri Johnson

Unlike the hot cocoa mix, running crystallized coffee through your sifter will make the sifter retain this flavor for a little while. To counteract this, you can simply mix with a fork in a bowl.

Ensure that the extract is well mixed into the nonfat dry milk before stirring in the sifted powdered sugar.

About Uncle Guy, the namesake of this mix. I am not sure he created the recipe, but having a cup of this on the old wooden deck brings him back. "Uncle" Guy Hohstadt was an amazing man who loved to play his guitar, have a drink at 5 o'clock, and enjoy a pot cookie before bed. He may have been just the singing forest ranger to some. To me, he's a legend of the Emerald Triangle. Having a cup of coffee with Guy was a privilege and he will be missed. We hope this recipe helps bring a great morning with family and friends. We know that we miss going to see Uncle Guy and knowing the coffee was always on. This is our way keeping that pot on for eternity in his memory.

We miss you Unc.

As he has passed on, we wanted to show you the namesake of this recipe.

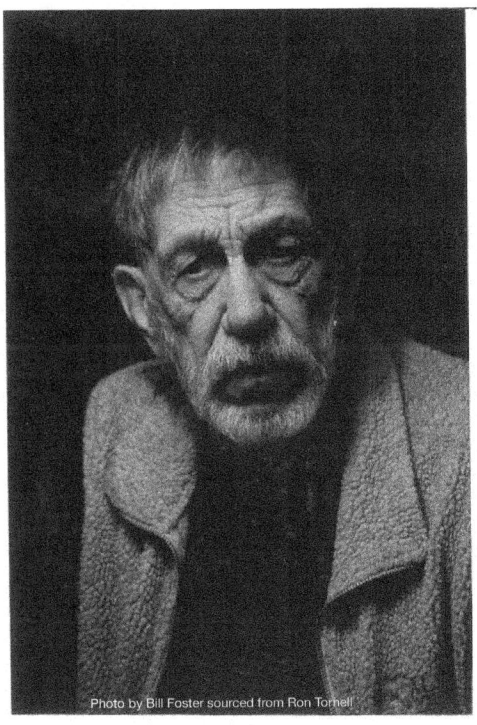

Photo by Bill Foster sourced from Ron Tornell

Lunch & Dinner

Cheeseburger

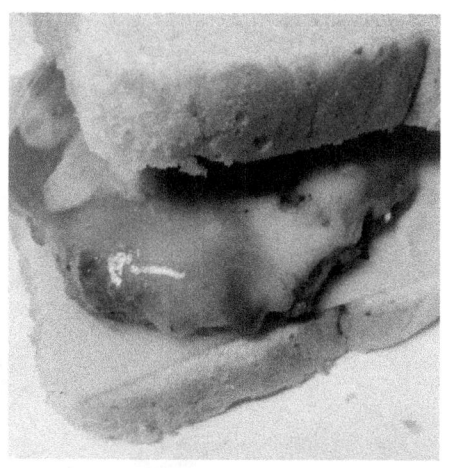

1 LB of ground meat

4 T butter

1 gram of dry ice extract

Burger fixins - onions, tomato slices, lettuce, cheese, and condiments

4 small hamburger buns or 4 Kaiser rolls

Salt and pepper

Prepare infused butter by adding dry ice extract to melted butter in a small bowl and stir. Let cool to spreadable butter.

Spread infused butter on bottom half of the 4 buns or rolls, and place in pan cooking over medium heat until toasted lightly.

Prepare meat into 4 patties, cooking until desired doneness. Sprinkle with desired salt and pepper. Add cheese while hot to allow for melting, if bread isn't prepared simultaneously, you can place the 4 cheese covered patties in the oven at 200 degrees to melt cheese.

Place warm burger patty on toasted bread and add fixins. Makes 4 burgers @ 250 mg.

We don't specify which type of meat with cheeseburgers as we enjoy most ground meat formed into patties. Experiment with chorizo, ground lamb, and even game meats to vary the flavors up a little. Dosage remains on the bun, so no loss to the grill from adding it directly to the meat.

Meatloaf

1 LB ground beef or 1/2 ground pork 1/2 ground sirloin

1/4 c Quick oats

Salt and pepper, to taste

1/2 LB cheddar cheese block, cubed

5 pieces of bacon

2 t minced garlic

Dash of smoked paprika

1 T Tabasco or Hot sauce

Ketchup, for topping

1 gram dry ice extract

Preheat oven to 350 degrees

Place meat in medium bowl, and sprinkle with extract evenly. Add all ingredients except bacon and ketchup into bowl and combine until ingredients are mixed well and easily hold loaf form. Push any exposed cheese block into loaf to avoid melting out into pan. Cut bacon in half to create 10 half pieces and lay them across the top of the loaf. Ketchup can then be drizzled over the top of the loaf to desired amount.

Place in preheated oven and bake until internal temperature reaches 150 degrees. Let rest 5 minutes before cutting, serves 4.

Meatball Sub

1/2 LB ground pork (plain or chorizo)

1/2 LB ground beef

1/2 c Italian breadcrumbs

1 jar marinara sauce, or 4 c homemade sauce

4 hoagie rolls

4 T butter

8 to 16 slices of cheese (Provolone or Mozzarella)

Parmesan cheese

1 t garlic, miced

1 gram dry ice extract or rosin concentrate

Infuse melted butter with extract and half of the garlic, let cool till spreadable. Preheat oven to 350 degrees.

Combine meat, breadcrumbs, and remaining garlic in a small bowl to create 24 small meatballs. Place on baking sheet, and cook in oven until internal temperature reaches 150 degrees. Add to medium saucepan with marinara and warm.

Spread 1 T of butter on each roll and evenly distribute cheese on bread. Add 6 meatballs to each roll, and sprinkle with parmesan heavily.

Each sandwich can be halved, and served to offer about 8 - 125 mg servings or you can serve whole for 4 - 250 mg servings.

Flatbread or Pizza

Pizza dough or flatbread(Any will do, and even gluten free will work here. Dough can be bought from any local pizza shop or handmade)

1/2 to 3/4 cup pizza sauce per pizza, homemade or canned of any style

1 or 2 c shredded cheese per pizza (premix or mixture of provolone, mozzarella, cheddar, and parmesan)

1/4 cup melted butter with 1 T garlic and a dash of parsley

Pizza Toppings

1 gram dry ice extract per pizza

As most of the recipes in this section will follow the normal recipe layout, This is more commercial. You can make as many pre-made pizzas as you like and freeze for up to 2 months. I also am vague on the sauce as you can use pesto, tomato, barbecue, or creamy garlic.

If you bought pizza skins (pre-rolled pizza dough from pizza shops or stores) you won't need to roll out the dough to about 1/8 of an inch thick and cut to 12 inch diameter pizzas. Skins are the industry term and are usually made when ordered. Stack floured skins with parchment to prevent sticking.

Add sauce to center of skin, and spread evenly to completely cover the skin. Add dry ice extract evenly across the pizza face. Add cheese evenly leaving 1 inch from the edge for a crust.

Place toppings, keeping precooked meats and greens below cheese and keeping uncooked meats for the final topping. In example if you wanted a supreme pizza you'd place in order: Sauce(tomato) and extract, cheese, 12 to 18 pepperoni, 8 salami, a handful of diced green peppers, 1/4 c mushrooms, 1/8 c olives, then 8 small balls of both Italian sausage and ground beef. Which is more work than a BBQ chicken pizza which is: Sauce(BBQ) and extract, bbq chicken meat, a handful of sliced onions, then cheese.

To cook a perfect cannabis pizza try not to weigh down the pizza with toppings. More food to process means your body will be to busy to process the THC into 11-hydroxy-metabolite.

You can cut skins to match vacuum sealable bags, place pizzas on parchment before sealing and freezing. Otherwise wrap with 2 layers of cling wrap (restaurant size rolls available at bulk stores)

Cooking directions are the same for ANY pizza regardless of the brand.

Preheat oven to 425 degrees

If you have a pizza stone, use it on the lowest oven rack.

Cook pizza for 12-15 minutes to desired crispiness of crust. Be sure to check at halfway and three quarters cooked to pop any bubbles in the crust with a fork.

Make sure any uncooked meat toppings have completely cooked. If extra cheese is desired add at last check for bubbles.

Let sit for 2 to 3 minutes before cutting.

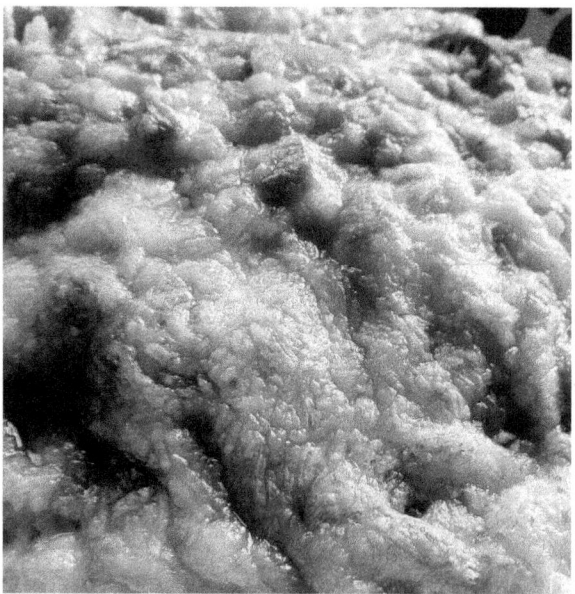

Edibles Mythology

Myth #3 Going to the club and buying an edible is the same thing as getting one off the street. They all sell the same things.

FALSE

No one on the street is required to maintain state regulated testing schedules. Also, the health department hasn't usually inspected the street dealers kitchen. Street edibles aren't exactly perfect on the dosing every time. Consistency will come with testing in labs. I trust lab tested edibles more, sorry.

DESSERTS

As we enter the dessert section, we want to point out that most desserts aren't made to entice children. Sweets, and other cakes or cookies have been used since the ancient times to make edible cannabis foods. Mahjoon, a nut butter infused with hashish or dry ice extract has been eaten in north Africa since the dawn of their tribes. Even today with the severe drug laws in Morocco, it is still available as seen by Anthony Bourdain in 2015.

I give you the dessert section as a starting point, and I need you to experiment. This is where you'll learn to shine as an edible maker.

Between chocolate, cookies, cakes, breads, ice cream, marshmallows. You can then define the edible you wish to market, or the dessert menu for your future cannabis restaurant.

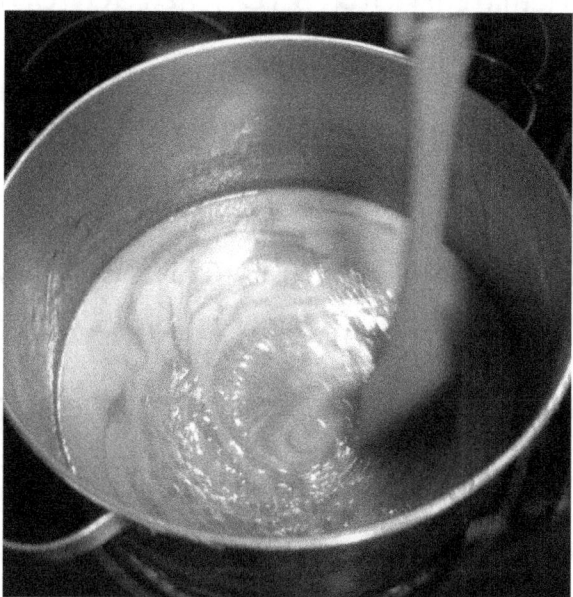

Homemade Marshmallows

These tasty morsels can be used in other recipes, or served covered in powdered sugar or dipped in infused chocolate. They are also a chance to learn how the extract can be added to heated sugar. Breaking the rules as most recipes require a fat or oil to bond it to. The sucrose crystals tend to carry the extract while making active the THC in the intense heat of the construction of cannabis candy. That's right, the extract can be added directly to caramel, taffy, and even suckers. It can even be bonded to regular sugar from alcohol infused with cannabis much like making colored sugar. We just haven't seen the industry use marshmallows, so we teach you using this interestingly missing product. Also I never see a marshmallow cereal treat recipe, so here you go.

3 pkgs unflavored gelatin

1 c ice cold water, divided

12 oz granulated sugar(approx 1 1/2 c)

1 c light corn syrup

1/4 t kosher salt

1 t vanilla extract

1/4 c confectioners sugar

1/4 c cornstarch

1.5 g dry ice extract for large, 3 g for smaller marshmallows

Nonstick Spray

Place gelatin into the bowl of a stand mixer along with 1/2 cup of the water. Have the whisk attachment ready.

In a small saucepan combine the remaining 1/2 cup water, granulated sugar, corn syrup and salt. Place over medium high heat, cover and allow to cook for 3 to 4 minutes. Uncover, clip a candy thermometer onto the side of the pan and continue to cook until the mixture reaches 240 degrees F, approximately 7 to 8 minutes. Once the mixture reaches this temperature add the dry ice extract, stir quickly and remove from heat.

Turn the mixer on low speed and, while running, slowly pour the sugar syrup down the side of the bowl into the gelatin mixture. Once you have added all the syrup, increase the speed to high. Continue to whip until the mixture becomes very thick and is lukewarm, approximately 12 to 15 minutes. Add the vanilla during the last minute of whipping. While the mixture is whipping prepare the pans as follows.

Here's where decisions need to be made, large or small marshmallows. Large is far more useful for dipping, desserts, or eating as a single treat. Smaller will be easier to toss into fruit salads, jello molds, and many other mass produceable edibles. These will probably be eaten as finger foods so be sure of the next step before you move.

For Large marshmallows: Combine the confectioners' sugar and cornstarch in a small bowl. Lightly spray a 13 by 9-inch metal baking pan with nonstick cooking spray. Add the sugar and cornstarch mixture and move around to completely coat the bottom and sides of the pan. Return the remaining mixture to the bowl for later use.

When ready, pour the mixture into the prepared pan, using a lightly oiled spatula for spreading evenly into the pan. Dust the top with enough of the remaining sugar and cornstarch mixture to lightly cover. Reserve the rest for later. Allow the marshmallows to sit uncovered for at least 4 hours and up to overnight.

Turn the marshmallows out onto a cutting board and cut into 1-inch squares using a pizza wheel dusted with the confectioners' sugar mixture. Once cut, lightly dust all sides of each marshmallow with the remaining mixture, using additional if necessary. Store in an airtight container good for a couple weeks.

For smaller marshmallows: Simply line 2 large baking sheets with parchment, spray with nonstick spray and dust with confectioners sugar and cornstarch mixture.

Load marshmallow mixture into a piping bag, and begin creating strips lengthwise using the 1/2 inch tip. Leaving about an inch between each row. Dust with confectioners mixture again. Let sit for 4 hours.

Dust kitchen shears with confectioners sugar mix and cut the strips every half inch. Dust lightly any edges not covered. Place in an airtight container. If not eaten within a week, drop into a batch of hot cocoa mix. The solidification will be stopped as the marshmallows will end up liquifying in the boiling water.

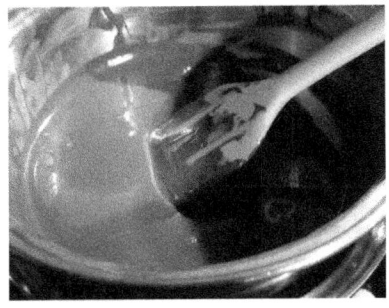

Making Chocolate

I am lucky enough to have gotten to spend time with the best of the best when it comes to cannabis infused chocolates. "Nibs" are an industry term for chocolate chips or melting chocolate discs from a friend overseas. I use all chocolate interchangeably, so as you see that term in the recipe. Know that nibs are a term for any chocolate pieces.

To do it you can choose either using nibs, or creating it from scratch. The later which is difficult does taste wonderful, is also far more time consuming than melting chocolate pieces or nibs and adding something to allow it to reconstitute without ruining it. The top edibles makers have been using this trick for years. Shortening added to melted bagged semisweet morsels or nibs also provides an amazing chocolate to dip macaroons or other food into and cooling back down. The chocolate will retain a silky smooth texture and look fantastic.

Try to keep your bars to about 200 milligrams of extract. Any more and taste becomes compromised. If you are planning on creating your own blend of chocolate try blending mixtures of dark and milk chocolate nibs. I like to add 15% dark to 85% milk to blend a particular flavor. I'd like you to keep in mind that these chocolate companies have done most of the work for you. Focus groups have refined their production to create a product that is not only well recognized. They have survived decades of trial by fire in the market to create the handful of major chocolate companies we have today.

For those in the mass production edible world, it's far easier to simply add a small amount of shortening to prepackaged nibs to create the desired consistency. For the purists, here's how to make mock chocolate from scratch:

1/2 c Cocoa powder

1/2 c cocoa butter

1/2 c coconut oil

1/3 to 1/2 cup honey, agave, or raw cane sugar

(Extract weight is dependent upon number of bars or treat being made. Keep bars to 200 mg each. Make dipping chocolate with 4 g extract and divide finished number of treats into 4000 for dosage level.)

Sift cocoa powder into a bowl, add the grated cocoa butter and oil to a warm bowl mix with a spoon to grind larger pieces of cocoa. Add to food processor and blend into a fine paste.

Heat water in a small pot till almost simmering, and add cocoa paste. Remove from heat, and add sweetener or sugar to taste. Return to food processor and pulse until all lumps are gone.

Add to mold, and chill till solid.

To really go the distance you'll need to ferment actual cocoa beans, and then get cocoa butter. Find that recipe, and just add the dry ice extract.

Bonus Recipes:

Buzz Bombs - Dip roasted coffee beans in melted chocolate and let cool, repeat until a thick layer of chocolate surrounds the bean. Some prefer dark chocolate for this.

Chocolate covered strawberries - Using large strawberries, available online or seasonally for your area. Dip and set on a parchment sheet to cool. Drizzle with dark chocolate for a festive treat.

Dip infused cookies for a double up on the THC.

Making Cookies

I am personally a cookie fan. Knowing that cookies are really all the same recipes with minor twists helps a lot. When I was in school, my home economics teacher let slip the base sugar cookie dough was the foundation for most of the famous cookies in the world.

Base tricks to creating the perfect cookie come from stores like cookie shops in the malls that remain nameless. Refrigerator dough makes good cookies, but frozen dough makes for a soft and crunchy cookie simultaneously. If you are using margarine, you'll have to at least chill the dough in the freezer.

Vegan and Gluten free cookies are also still wonderful. I know that some of these types of foods could be considered bland. Thankfully you can add flavors from strains like Chocolope for chocolate chip cookies or Pineapple and Mango also improve on lemon drop cookies. My only failure was with a strawberry cheesecake cookie, so know that sometimes the experiments fail. My interest lies in creating the perfect dose and size while hiding all the negative flavors sometimes perceived by consumers.

Basic sugar cookie (or basic refrigerator cookie dough):

1/3 c butter or margarine

1/3 c shortening

3/4 c sugar

1 t baking powder

1 egg

1 t vanilla

2 c AP Flour

3.5 g dry ice extract

Cream together butter, extract, and shortening in mixer bowl. Add sugar in slowly until creamed well. Add baking powder and a dash of salt. Scrape down bowl, add 2/3 flour and continue mixing. After dough begins forming, add remaining flour. Divide dough once formed, and chill for at least 3 hours. Roll out 1/2 on lightly floured surface till 1/8 inch thick. Cut and cook at 350 degrees (375 for crispy) for 8 to 10 minutes or until edges brown. Makes 36 cookies.

Additional candy pieces can be added including candy covered chocolates, crushed peppermint candy, and even some chunks of candy bars. I would say you can turn it into chocolate chip cookies but you'll need a slightly different recipe.

Chocolate Chip Cookies

1/2 c shortening

1/2 c butter

1/2 c sugar

1 c packed brown sugar

1/2 t baking soda

2 eggs

1 t vanilla

2 1/2 c AP flour (or 1 1/2 c AP flour and 1 c cake flour)

2 c semisweet chocolate chips

3 g dry ice extract for 50 mg / 6 g extract for 100 mg

[optional nuts of your favorite variety just add 1 1/2 c]

Cream sugar, butter, shortening, eggs, and vanilla. Sift flour, baking powder and divide. Add 1/2 of dry ingredients to creamed mixture and beat until smooth. Add remaining flour and chocolate pieces (also nuts) mix until dough forms. Drop it in rounded spoonfuls onto baking sheet. Bake at 350 for 8 to 10 minutes. Makes 60 cookies.

Large cookies - Bake at 375 for 11 to 13 minutes. Makes about 20 cookies.

Bars - Press dough into un-greased 15x10x1 pan. Bake at 375 for 15 to 20 minutes. Makes 48 bars

Additional candy pieces, chocolate chunks, and variations can be made(i.e.-white chocolate macadamia nut, or cocoa powder for chocolate-chocolate chip)

Making Ice Cream

Very simply Ice cream can be infused, but requires the same minor preparation. You need cannabis infused milk. For every 2 quarts of ice cream, you'll need 4 cups infused milk

To accurately hit the correct dosing, you'll need 1.6 grams of extract. Making it about 50 mg per dose in 1/2 cup of ice cream.

So when the recipe calls for infused milk. Prepare milk in saucepan and bring to simmer, stir in extract, and cool in fridge. Viola, you have infused milk.

The basic recipe for ice cream hasn't changed. To make it easier, buy an ice cream mixer/freezer. This will prevent you from losing you mind stirring the slowly freezing mixture by hand.

Vanilla Ice Cream

4 cups infused milk (half &half, or light cream may be used)

1 1/2 c sugar

1 T vanilla

2 c heavy whipping cream

Mix well, and pour into ice cream maker. Use machine for alloted period, remove dasher, cover with top or wax paper. Freeze (or ripen) for four hours, and enjoy.

Chocolate Ice Cream - Reduce sugar to 1 cup, add 16 oz chocolate syrup

Coffee Ice Cream - When infusing milk or half and half add 2 to 3 Tablespoons of instant coffee.

Cherries, candy, and other additives can be to your wildest dreams. If you've ever been to a Cold Stone Creamery you understand what I mean.

Fruit Ice Creams - Remove vanilla, Add 1 cup fresh or frozen fruit of your choice.

Chocolate Velvet Ice Cream - 4 cups infused heavy cream, 1 1/3 c condensed milk, 1 16 oz can chocolate syrup, 2/3 cup finely chopped nuts of choice.

Making Cakes and Breads

Your big trick on this one is sifting the dry ice extract into the flour as you begin the recipe process. That means that you can technically sift the extract with cake mixes as well. Try to avoid any prepackaged cakes or bread mixes that have fruit or other solids like confetti cakes.

The other trick is to substitute duck eggs for chicken eggs. Duck eggs have been shunned by many people for little or no reason. They are a little more expensive, but make any cake or bread quite a bit better upon rising. Chefs can argue this, but when making cannabis food it does help.

I am a huge fan of Harriet's Cake, which is a chocolate cake with a melted tub of chocolate frosting poured over. This is so rich it completely hides the taste of cannabis regardless of dosing.

Pineapple upside down cakes, and other fruit cakes are also good choices for infusion. One of the great parts about cakes and breads are the shelf life. You can freeze breads and cakes for extended periods to thaw and decorate as necessary.

The cupcake is huge in the edibles world as the dosing is easy, and you know how much to eat. I've found friends in delirium after eating half a pan of cake and not realizing the huge amount of cannabis they ingested.

Yellow Cake

2 1/2 c AP flour

2 1/2 t baking powder

1/2 t salt

2/3 c butter

1 3/4 c sugar

1 1/2 t vanilla

2 duck eggs, beaten till aerated and light yellow

1 1/4 c milk

1.2 g dry ice extract

Grease and flour a 13x9 pan.

Combine dry ingredients except sugar in a bowl, set aside. Whip butter in a bowl with mixer for 30 seconds. Add sugar and vanilla and continue with mixer until it becomes a light mixture. Add eggs in slowly, then dry mixture and milk alternately till combined.

Bake at 375 degrees about 33 minutes or until a toothpick comes out clean. Cool on wire rack. Makes enough for 12 pieces at about 100 mg per serving.

Cupcakes - fill paper lined muffin trays to about half full, or use a mini cupcake tray and measuring cup to create about 30 regular cupcakes. Bake at 375 for 18 to 20 minutes. As always the toothpick is the best test.

Citrus Cake - add 2 t finely ground orange or lemon peel to batter.

Marble Cake - By melting 1 cup chocolate pieces of choice in microwave and adding 3 T melted butter and 1 1/2 c powdered sugar and 3 T hot water. You can mix this well and pour the melted chocolate over the cake in it's pan after cooling. Creating the marble cake we all love. Also can be double infused as the chocolate pieces can be tainted as well.

Chocolate Chip Cake - add 1/2 package of semisweet morsels after batter is in the pan.

Confetti Yellow Cake - Add 2 T candy sprinkles during the last 20 seconds of mixing.

Other great additions to the cake include adding 1/2 c chocolate syrup to 1/3 of the batter. Add the chocolate bater to the top of the remaining batter. Adding 1 1/2 T instant coffee to the batter for a great coffee dessert cake.

You can also add a teaspoon of your favorite extract like root beer, maple, or even 1 cup of your favorite fruit syrup. These will all add amazing changes to a very basic recipe.

The dry ice extract can be easily added to the creamed butter and sugar of any homemade cake recipe. This extract will also allow you to add it to the flour of depression cakes and other foods that don't use butter or shortening. My friends who want to use coconut oil or butter are welcome to simply replace it. For the people at high altitude cannabis doesn't change your elevation needs. You'll have to do your basic additions or adjustments.

Snacks

Sweet and Spicy Sriracha Cash-ews

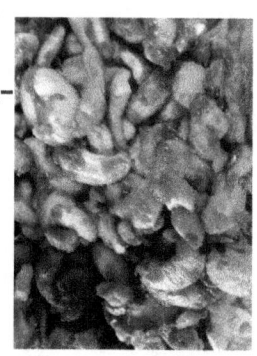

1/2 cup packed light brown sugar

2 Tablespoon Sriracha sauce

1 inch piece of fresh ginger, finely grated or 1/4 t ground ginger

3 cups cashews

1 t crushed red pepper

3 g dry ice extract

Preheat the oven to 350 degrees

In small pan over medium heat, combine brown sugar, Sriracha sauce, and ginger, stirring frequently until the sugar melts (about 5 minutes).Remove from heat.

Pour cashews into mixing bowl. Drizzle the sugar mixture over the cashews and stir well to evenly coat them.

Spread the cashews out on baking sheet and bake until crispy (about 15-20 minutes), stirring about every 5 minutes (stir at least twice). Note: to prevent cashews from sticking line a baking sheet with parchment paper or silicone mat.

Sriracha Bark - Add 1 cup of finished cashews to a sheet of melted chocolate till at desired thickness on a sheet of parchment paper or silicone. Break and serve.

Cracked and Jacked - Add to a batch of caramel corn with a chance to double up by infusing the caramel corn recipe as well. It makes the favorite sweet salty treat from childhood seem like it's grown up a little.

NOTE: This recipe can be made with simple ground up cannabis. I've had some great success with just adding 2 grams of ground flower.

Grammie Annes Candied Nuts

3 c raw or roasted cashews, peanuts, whole almonds, or pecan halves (Mixed to your preference)

1 c sugar

4 T butter

1 t vanilla

2.5 g dry ice extract

Line a baking sheet with foil, or use a silicone mat. Butter and set aside.

In a 10 inch cast iron skillet, combine ingredients and cook over a medium high heat. Shake skillet, do not stir. As sugar begins to melt turn heat to low. Continue cooking until sugar is golden brown. While on low, stir occasionally.

Pour on prepared baking sheet, and let cool.

Break and serve. Makes about 20 oz (24 servings at about 100 mg per serving.

Beef Jerky

The next two recipes in the book require either learning to operate your oven as a dehydrator, or buying an affordable food making tool. We have and use the dehydrator semi regularly for dried fruit. This is one of two ways to take advantage of rare edibles like infused beef jerky and fruit roll ups for adults

2 lbs flank steak

Brine:

2/3 c Worcestershire sauce

2/3 c soy sauce

1 T honey

2 t freshly ground black pepper

2 t onion powder

1 t liquid smoke

1 t red pepper flakes

1/2 t Spanish style smoked paprika

Final coating:

2 g dry ice extract

3 T teriyaki, barbecue, or hot sauce

Trim steak. I ask my butcher to do this for me, they are usually happy to help. Bag and place in the freezer for 1 to 2 hours to firm it up.

Cut along the grain. Cut thin for sheet jerky, but if you want your jerky in casings as they sell most beef sticks. You'll need to grind and inject into your own casings at home. More equipment, more time preparing, but to each their own.

Place meat along with all the remaining brine ingredients into a large, 1-gallon plastic zip-top bag and molest with prejudice. Refrigerate for at least 4 hours.

Remove meat, pat dry, Place evenly across baking sheet, and brush with final coating across one side of all pieces, if final coating remains flip meat as you move it and coat the other side of the jerky. Move dehydrator trays on to machine.

Follow dehydrator instructions till finished. Store in a cool dry place for up to 3 months.

1/8 of finished weight should be about 250 mg.

Note: Jerky is like chili, you can make it however it pleases you. I am well versed in different manufacturers making recipe books that come with their product. You must add the final coating to whatever jerky you make. The brine is a poor carrier, and you simply waste the product unless added to the outer glaze on the jerky.

Dehydrated Fruit Strips

Most dehydrators come with a recipe for fruit leather, or as I grew up calling them fruit roll ups. Here's the thing, I like them as edibles due to shelf life, taste, and easy dosing.

Fruit Puree

Plastic wrap

1 g of dry ice extract per tray of fruit leathers approximately

Follow manufacturers instructions, while pureeing fruit sprinkle in dry ice extract. Add to trays and let dehydrate.

Cut into 1/8 of the round or square depending on dehydrator shape. Wrap tightly in plastic wrap.

Each cut strip should be about 125 mg each. Good for 6 months if refrigerated in vacuum sealed bags.

Super powered strips - Add mango to any fruit puree to increase THC absorption. Mango has a compounding reaction that works even after the drying process. Mango doesn't have to be overpowering, just in the mix.

Mango Madness Leather - Using a puree of mango, pineapple pulp, tangerine pulp, and dragonfruit. Do not add tangerine or pineapple juice as the puree will be too moist for a good leather. Separate by using a juicer that strains the pulp.

Popcorn Recipes

Party Popcorn

6 c popped popcorn

2 T butter

2 T parmesan cheese

> And/or

1 T macaroni and cheese powder (any flavor powder)

> Or

1 t Taco seasoning or 1/2 t cayenne powder

1 T finely chopped chives or parsley (optional)

1.2 g dry ice extract

Tossed warm popcorn in a large bowl with butter. Immediately toss in parmesan, or other choice of topping. Sprinkle dry ice extract evenly and continue tossing.

If desired add parsley or chives.

Toss again to coat evenly and serve. Six servings at about 200 mg each.

Caramel Corn

8 c popped popcorn

3/4 c packed brown sugar

6 T butter

3 T light corn syrup

1/4 t baking soda

1/4 t vanilla

1.4 g dry ice extract

Remove unpopped kernels from popcorn. Put popcorn in roasting pan. Cover a baking sheet in foil and butter, set aside. In a saucepan over medium heat bring brown sugar, corn syrup, and butter to a boil. Without stirring, boil for 5 minutes at a moderate heat. Remove from heat and add extract, vanilla, and baking soda. Stir well, and pour syrup mixture over popcorn. Gently toss to coat. Bake at 350 degrees for 20 minutes (stir at 15 minutes). Spread caramel corn on foil to cool. Store in an airtight container. Makes 7 servings of 200 mg.

Popcorn Balls

18 c popped popcorn

2 c sugar

1 c water

1/2 c light corn syrup

1 t vinegar

1/2 t salt

1 T vanilla

2 g dry ice extract

Remove all unpopped popcorn. Place in greased roasting pan and keep in a 300 degree oven while making candy portion.

Butter the sides of a 2 quart saucepan. Combine sugar, water, corn syrup, vinegar, and salt.

Cook over medium high heat and bring to a boil. Stir to dissolve all sugar, and bring to a boil. Attach candy thermometer, bring heat to medium. Keep at a moderate temp while boiling until mixture reaches 250, stirring occasionally.

When it's ready, remove heat and add extract and vanilla. Stir to combine well. Slowly pour and stir into popcorn lightly. Once cool enough to handle, form into balls with buttered hands. Makes about 20 balls at 100 mg per ball. You can also roll in green sugar, while cooling, to mark as infused.

Sauces

Heavenly Hot Sauce

20 Tabasco or serrano chiles, stemmed and cut crosswise into 1/8 inch slices, or 12 very ripe red jalapenos (about 10 oz), or 15 Habanero peppers (also 10 oz)

1 3/4 T minced garlic

3/4 c thin sliced onions

3/4 t salt

1 t vegetable or sunflower oil

2 c water

1 c white vinegar

4 g dry ice extract

Cook the peppers, garlic, onions, salt and oil in a non-reactive saucepan over high heat. Saute for 3 minutes. Add the water and continue to cook, stirring occasionally, for about 20 minutes, or until peppers are very soft and almost all the liquid has evaporated. (Note: this should be done in a very well-ventilated area! Otherwise it's a lot like being pepper sprayed.)

Remove from heat, cool to room temperature. In a food processor, process the mixture for 15 to 20 seconds, or until smooth. With the food processor running, add the vinegar through the feed tube. Then season with more salt, if necessary. (This will depend on the heat level as well as the vinegar used.) Strain the mixture through fine mesh, and transfer to sterilized pint jar or bottle. If shelving the jar or bottle should be canned correctly.

Dosage with be different depending on how much used.

Avoid using for at least a couple weeks as the mixture will need time for the flavors to correctly age. Can be stored for about 6 months without canning for later use. The higher the heat, the less the extract will be tasted. Heat, especially super hot peppers, hide most of the cannabis tastes, and most other tastes as well. You've been warned.

Badass Barbecue Sauce

1 c Ketchup

1/2 c water

1 T dried minced onion

1/4 cup vinegar

1 T sugar

1 T Worcestershire sauce

1/4 t salt

1/4 t celery seed

1/4 t hot pepper sauce

2 T prepared mustard

1/4 t garlic powder

4 g dry ice extract

Add all ingredients to a saucepan, and bring to a boil. Reduce heat and simmer uncovered for 15 minutes or desired consistency.

Brush on meats, cooking for another 10 minutes on grill or as a roast.

Makes about 2 cups of sauce. Use as a dipping sauce for your favorite food as a condiment to get the best dosing results. I tend to store them in 2 ounce containers to eat with chicken strips.

Hot Barbecue Sauce - Add 1/2 t chili powder, 1/2 t cayenne powder, and 1/2 t dried crushed red pepper.

Carolina Style Barbecue Sauce - Add 2 T apple cider vinegar or a little more until desired taste and consistency. Carolina sauces tend to be thinner, and have a brighter bite to them. You can also add more hot pepper sauce for flavor.

Emerald Triangle Ranch Dressing

1 clove garlic, minced

1/4 t kosher salt

1 c mayonnaise

1/2 c sour cream

1/4 c Italian flat-leaf parsley leaves, minced

2 T fresh dill, minced

1 T minced fresh chives

1 t Worcestershire sauce

1/2 t ground black pepper

1/2 t white vinegar

1/4 t smoked paprika

1/8 teaspoon cayenne pepper

Dash hot sauce

1/4 to 1/2 c buttermilk (as needed for desired consistency)

Sprinkle salt on minced garlic and mash it into a paste with a fork. Combine remaining ingredients into a bowl. Add the buttermilk to desired consistency and mix to combine, tasting frequently and adjusting seasonings as needed. Chill for a couple of hours, overnight for best results. Thin using a little more buttermilk.

Spicy Ranch - Add 1 T taco seasoning, and a few dashes of hot sauce.

Green Goddess Dressing - Add 1/2 an avocado and pulse in a food processor.

Garlic Lovers Ranch - Increase garlic amount to 2 1/2 minced cloves.

All dressings can be tainted, this is just my favorite. Italian dressing and Caesar are also good choices to infuse.

Chillin' Chocolate Sauce

I want to be the one who gets to explain the easy way, and the hard way for this. You can easily cheat this recipe by simply adding dry ice extract directly to the store bought sauces and warming them to 180 for a few seconds to bond the extract. I have added a little water if the sauce seems to become too thick, but more nibs usually helps.

This chocolate sauce isn't the kind you add to milk for chocolate milk. It's definitely more on the hot fudge side. Normally you wouldn't need to say this. I already was able to see people complaining about how thick it was and how it wouldn't combine well with milk. The time saver for that syrup is the same for cheating this sauce, bring to 180 in a pan and evenly spread the extract. Stir till cool. Bottle and use on ice cream, in milkshakes, warmed and drizzled, or as an ingredient in molten chocolate cakes.

1 1/2 c semisweet nibs

1/2 c butter

1 1/3 c sugar

1 1/3 c evaporated milk

7 g dry ice extract

Melt nibs and butter in a medium size heavy pot. Once completely melted, stir in sugar. Gradually add evaporated milk over low heat. Bring to a gentle boil and hold for 8 minutes. Continue stirring vigorously as you remove from heat. Cool and transfer into 2 pint canning jars. Makes 3 cups sauce.

Peanut Butter Cup Sauce - Add 1/2 c smooth or crunchy peanut butter

Dark Forest Raspberry Sauce - Exchange nibs for: 1/2 c semisweet, 1 c dark and add 1/4 to 1/2 c ripe raspberries.

Buzz Bomb* Sauce - Add 1 T instant coffee crystals and optionally you can switch all nibs to dark.

*-Named *after the candy I loved as a seventeen year old: buzz bombs, or the more commonly seen dark chocolate covered espresso beans. Description is the ingredient list.*

The Green Rush, The Federal Law, and The Actual Price of Weed

My Experience So Far In The Rush

I've been lucky enough to spend a few months working the trim circuit in the Emerald Triangle. It makes it easier to find one of those jobs when you are related to, or are friends with a local. So don't expect to just up and move there and find work. The season I worked, was towards the end of the rush there. Many more states ended up adding medical programs soon after that, and some even went full legal. In 2016 we have four states and Washington, DC with recreational marijuana. Several more, including my home state of Nevada, are considering legalization as well. This is sending ripple effects through what was once a thriving black market, and medical markets as well.

The multitude of access is providing thousands of once fearful users. Unique access to this plant. With recreational and markets taking on the prices of the once prominent black market. The cartels, and anyone once propped up by the illegal market. Are now finding the competition to be better at beating their price points.

With less dangers, as the current administration is supposed to be curbing federal intervention into the states that have decided to legalize cannabis. We still find raids happening. Just not as high on the media radar. Patients in several states are still being raided by local law enforcement for various reasons. The folks in law enforcement will still arrest you, or take your weed. Some police lately have been known to just ask you to dump it if you can't produce a medical card (or just don't have one). Some police will even refuse to return medicine, even though your state allows medical cannabis. Many police officers are even willing to completely ignore it. This is something I praise officials for. Just don't expect it to happen to you.

Here's where my thoughts on the subject of jobs and the cannabis industry may help you. With these new markets, come new jobs. I understand the draw. I too would love to have a position in the industry other than this narration. I would love to be able to say my whole world revolved around cannabis. This would be my favorite career move of all time. I have had friends move to the legal states, and have even been offered jobs designing grow environments in Colorado. The more access to cannabis, the more likely to find a cannabis job. Just don't bet on this blindly, please make sure the job is yours before you go moving there. If you plan on waiting for the rush to hit you (like I am). You may be waiting multiple years on this plan. If this is your long term goal, try to get in to help define the medical and recreational regulations. This may also help you gain access to others in the industry already. This can lead to later employment with someone who may value your skills.

Please do everyone a favor, and market yourself well. Any thoughts of that parody stoner making it big. Are false, and your actions will scare off any employer. Being clean cut, having a proper image, and being personable will be your way in. Don't expect a grower position immediately, you may need to pull a Drake. Starting from the bottom sucks, but it will teach you humility. The only way you are getting that prized upper tier cannabis position, is knowing someone on the inside of the operation.

I know it sucks to hear that. It's not something I like telling people. It's the truth though. If your goal is one of those jobs. You are going to need to start a full company with your own backers. It is to be hoped that soon there will be a Pot Shark Tank, or Pot Crowdfunding. That way more of us can feature our skills; to the stoners with the capital to invest in the truly talented cannabis entrepreneurs out there.

If you are doing a job search, make sure and tailor your resume. Cannabis industry employers are quite aware that there isn't much in the way of checking your trimmer and cannabis use history. In fact, that isn't really the thing they are looking for.

Industry employers are searching for trustworthy, honest, friendly individuals. Any history of this should be helpful. If you work in a big box store, get your supervisor to write a letter of recommendation on your trustworthiness. If you look at what you do, you can find places where these traits appear. Your coworkers or another good reference should be willing to vouch for you, if not, you may need to work on being more employable altogether before trying to break into this industry.

There are several schools to help train you to be better prepared for employment in the cannabis world. If you are like me, you may find it to be very basic. They may cover some of the topics necessary to become a budtender, or some other basic industry job. Cooking classes will cover most of the same things you will learn by simply spending some time researching extractions, and watching all the episodes of Good Eats. This will save you a few thousand on courses. If you really have an in depth question. Any edible maker should be willing to answer it, if not just ask a favorite local chef (omit cannabis if you feel uncomfortable).

I am quite upset at the lack of industry positions in some of the less populated states like Nevada and Arizona. The jobs become similar to an old boys network, or rich guys club. Your searches will end in interview after interview, and no calls back. People can try to say I'm wrong. I can simply point out the truth. The price of the licenses of operation, lack of patient resale, and the necessary liquid capital. Make it so the little patient or edible maker, can never make it to the table with these people. In Nevada, over a hundred licenses were provisionally granted. These operations then began to open, and they made sure that only Las Vegas would have the bulk of the licenses. These people are also deciding to gouge the patients while they still can. Not only by digging into their pocketbook, but they are limiting the milligrams on edibles to a 100 mg maximum medical dose.

The goal of some of these folks is to get as much money as possible, before they have to drop the price of the weed to the real price. I don't know where you are right now. In all reality, it doesn't matter where you are. The widespread influx of growers nationwide means the value of cannabis is far less than you'd believe. Even after the lights, nutrients, trimmers, packaging, and transportation.

Is cannabis destined to be the next tulip?

If you haven't read about tulip-mania and the negative effects on the involved economies. You're in for a shock as to the artificial value some people can place on flowers. Let's get to bottom of it without prejudice.

The actual value of cannabis is between $1200 and $1600 a pound. You can argue with me until you are blue in face. I and many thousands of other growers have grown cup quality medicine for that actual value. The prices people are paying are all based on the old black market model. This value is inflated due to illegality and hands in the operations. If the cannabis comes from a legal source, and sun grown medicine is allowed. The supply can (and does) become flooded in fall and should send the price of medicine down drastically.

With some states using indoor only models, and new localized regulations coming in to play removing access to sun grown medicine. They are now quietly feeding the energy companies a kick back for energy use by growers. This will also create a limited access to patients in 2017. As most outdoor growers are not interested in buying expensive greenhouses that draw attention. They also may not end up repaying their initial investments as the market begins to slowly drop. They aren't worried about cops or feds, they're worried about thieves willing to do almost anything to steal crops. Also, they dread the insect problems, as most sun grows never really see. The types of possible infestations and problems involved indoor and hydroponics. I've seen growers that stripped down like a hazmat operation and completely scrubbed to prevent carrying mites, stray pollen, or molds from the outside world in.

The legal storefronts, clubs, and collectives all want you to believe the artificially inflated price of $3600-$6000 per pound. If you lived through the great recession. You'll understand what I would call a "cannabis bubble". This is fueling an artificial peak in the price of this garden weed. The problem with this bubble, is that the government got a taste in most cases. So they are now worried about the price tumbling too quickly. The taxes they enjoy now, are going to drop like lead bars off a table. Crashing back down to the real value.

The day cannabis became legal in Colorado, the street price of cannabis went from about $150 an ounce for top shelf medical grade flowers. To a wasteland of nothing on the black market. When I say that, I mean that most dealers just quit. Illegal growers stopped their Colorado operations, packing up and moving to places better suited for black market sales. Or doing what most people did, they went back to regular workforce jobs and just quit dealing.

This fact should mean something to you. It means that the market is based on a commodity valued at 400+% over its real value. When something isn't realistically valued, the market for it is going to face steep drops soon. Remember the price of your home back in 2007? Compare it to that and then after the bubble burst in say 2008 or 2009. That is what I mean by a cannabis bubble. This is a financial bubble, we should preemptively pop as an industry. To make the same amount of money, the industry will have to produce more. Not something we should let suddenly happen on a random October day in the near future.

I know it may be hard to hear it, but we can afford to make less. Too many patients need access, and many need large quantities to create oil. The industry leaders should see the benevolence in these actions. Taking the high road, no pun intended, and taking it on the chin. This will allow for the realistic growth of the market, and provide the ability for amateur and expert crops and products. Providing the needed range in prices, and allowing for the poorest patients to get good quality medicine at fair prices.

The price you pay is due to many hands in the cookie jar. First, the regulators are getting their cut with the licensing, and paperwork. They also take in the patient licensing, so we are talking about quite a bit of money in the grand scale. Next, The labs in Nevada are getting a pretty penny. As California lab testing dropped down to an $80 testing fee for anyone. Nevada is running at $700 per test, testing every 5 pounds (and patients can't even test their homegrown). So, if a harvest pulls 20.25 pounds. The cultivator has to pay $2800 for testing on 4 batches of the same cannabis, and destroys the quarter pound (a complete waste) to not have to pay more than the cannabis is worth to test it. These fees and costs all get passed on to the patient. Giving us the black market again, only it's lining the pockets of he rich and powerful and called state sanctioned.

To do this at an accelerated rate, we also need the federal government to reclassify the schedule 1 drug. Maybe moving off scheduling altogether. OK, that would be dreaming really big. You're never gonna get there if you don't dream it now. Without that, we will never see a financial acceptance. Making banking easier, and helping provide safer environments for the money that we've all seen accumulate. Law enforcement will then have to drop the facade. Making everything safer as the whole system shifts over to complete legal use.

It's not impossible to imagine. The day they stop this war, we see the beginnings of the end to fear. Commercial operations can enter the free market. Some say we will see the big box weed stores come in and ruin it all. I for one, think we will see a huge industry begin to blossom like the flowers that power it.

The Federal Position On Cannabis, May Be Over A Barrel

"The truth is like poetry, and people fucking hate poetry..."

-Overheard in a DC bar.

Politicians have the luxury of changing their minds as their constituents make their voices heard. Except on the position of legalizing marijuana. I've heard many officials quickly jump on the facts about our younger generations arrest records regarding cannabis. I have one, my family members have them, even my grandfathers dead brother grew illegally in Humboldt County long before I was born. Also long before the trend was to get that prized crop from the triangle. I hope that one of them legislatively succeeds with striking all cannabis arrests from everyones records. I would love to strike that bullshit misdemeanor from my record. Let's see them do it, I won't be holding my breath. I am writing this during the Sanders campaign of 2016. He may be the best option available so far. I won't presume to judge his chances of becoming president with many months left. So, let me just hope he gets it and legalizes cannabis like the government of Canada is supposedly doing.

If you think the DEA and other law enforcement are going to go quietly. You've lost your damn mind. They will go out and will try to take as much down as possible until then. The officials in California have shown that to be true. The DEA has pushed more raids through since Obama took office. The cops in Arizona raided Gregg Lendovski. A very sick patient, who was quietly treating himself with Simpson oil. I have seen some law enforcement offices slow the fearmongering, but most are still going in the same prohibitionist direction. The actions are those of people trying to save their own jobs. We know from numbers that if all the other drugs combined are the focus of police. Their budget will be far too little without the money used for marijuana prohibition.

The real reason that your officials can't seem to regulate cannabis. Is their complete lack of compassion for our individual situations. With a few exceptions like former Gov. Gary Johnson who has held a medical recommendation. Most politicians have no idea what it means to have to be a round the clock cannabis patient. They don't know what it means to be without your medicine after the year supply is used up. They don't know what it's like to not be able to afford to buy medicine from clubs because they are just too poor. They don't know how hard you've struggled to get to here. Therefore, your struggles don't really matter to them. Honestly, they have no use for your struggle because it won't get them reelected. If you weren't sure yet, they get quite a salary once elected. Something no elected official likes losing. Hey, we all know that money is the backdrop to everything. It's not reality or compassion in most cases.

If you can be involved in regulation creation. Please do your part to make everything in the patients favor. Making things more difficult for sick people just seems criminal to me.

As states create legal cannabis, you really need to be involved in their creation of regulations. I am more than happy to add a cap to the milligrams available to random people on the recreational market. Not so much when it comes down to patients. These are going to be things in your control if you get enough backing and public support. I hope to one day see a state with no plant limits per person. Then the markets and products introduced become matters of skill sets. Each person can have the chance to shine and really participate in the next true green rush.

One of the things people forget to think about with the legalization of cannabis. Comes with it, the legal hemp market. Outdoor commercial hemp can and will remove the cartels from our national forests out west. I know that sounds like a big jump but let me explain.

Cartels and illegal growers on national forest lands are there due to the remote awesome locations and conditions, and lack of wild male cannabis pollen. Introducing hemp into the rotations out west will create huge clouds of male pollen that will destroy any chance of seedless marijuana. Without good product to compete with the legal market, the cartels will move on to more profitable activities. The lack of willingness to change the laws is propping up their illegal activities. Showing again that law enforcement wants to continue prosecuting users and growers, and growers want the market to remain illegal to keep their illegal product quality high. All this work is a washout if legal hemp is allowed to create giant drifting clouds of low THC pollens that travel hundreds of miles in high winds. The next generation of seeds is now lowered THC, all the phenotypes are going to be different, and no consistency will be present in the following genetic hybrids. Very similar to trying to grow apples from the seeds inside, you'll likely not get a matching fruit tree to the seed. You'll probably get a cider apple that looks different and tastes different.

If the government doesn't know that fact. They are either stupid, or lying to you. Spain has a wild cannabis population, and the weather covers cannabis pollen counts. Meteorologists can talk using the internet, and we can see pictures and video online that will confirm my statements. This also destroys their statement that cannabis is getting stronger in potency as well. With wild pollen the THC will begin to slowly drop back down on some stable outdoor varieties after multiple seasons in the pollen. That is a theory, and until we can see it firsthand it will remain a theory.

You can help change things, regardless of what you think about politicians. Run for office, get in there and change things. You don't have to do much more than pay the fee to run unless you want to. I've even heard of people winning elections without even knocking on doors, making signs, or having meet and greets.

If you feel like this may never be legal, you are not alone. I've had periods where I've felt like the government would much rather us die than legalize a harmless plant. Just look at the brighter side, and enjoy the many legal states and many more coming online as time goes on. It's only a matter of time as Dr. Grinspoon says. The world will change, and we will move on from this prohibition. We all need to do our part to cull it.

The Cup, and The Income Gap

Cannabis cups can also provide good intelligence on the market and some great tastes to boot. The problem I have with the cups, and especially the High Times cup competitions. Is that the amount of free product you have to produce, and then also paying an entry fee. To then possibly have spent multiple thousands of dollars to come away empty handed. Seems to be a competition for those growers that have extra income they can just blow. Sometimes that means the quality may not be the best in the area. Just the best that could afford to participate. Feel free to reverse engineer anything they declare a winner. It's made from the same ingredients you have access to. The winning edible the past few years has been made in the kitchen the following weekend. Jerky comes out amazeballs, you're gonna also love making macaroons and other cookies once you perfect them for your dose and taste.

They do present the competitors with huge advertising opportunity. If you place, or even get an honorable mention. Your following will be boosted and will grow at an exponential rate. This can also provide celebrities with the chance to plug your products. Just don't think you'll have it all happen because you go compete. Many walk away unheard of, and out quite a lot of cash.

I've also had some amazing edibles from random companies that were quite tasty. The income gap that prevents these chefs from being recognized. Is shameful, and shows the rich get to participate. While the poor and sometimes underfunded have to just deal with being spectators. This is not limited to the edibles category. Flower, concentrates, and CBD categories are all subject to these income disparities as well.

Maybe one day there will be more even competition that includes the lower income bracket. Until then, we'll all have to just watch the rich people have their cannabis cup and corner the markets. I think that may be the only way we see a more diverse market and competition scene. I also see the future competitions using far more lab details than just personal choices. The stronger strains losing to flavor based judgements. As the turpenes are now helping define future strain combinations more than just THC content and visual profile of the flowers.

Without a change to this side of the industry. We will find more monopolies and gouging people. As the rich will be able to far surpass the growth of any startup. Since the cannabis industry startup isn't able to just go out and get a loan from the bank to help pay for cannabis competition costs. This seems to be an out of pocket kind of thing. I don't foresee an extra $6000 this year, let alone the next decade. That leaves me, and many others like me, with no chance of being able to compete in a cannabis cup.

Tools, Books, And Final Thoughts

Tools

I wanted to give you a basic list of tools if you plan on getting into edibles. Some of the stuff you are going to need before getting started on your edibles journey. Here's a short list:

- Scales, accurate ones and make sure you have all 3 sizes. Pound scale, gram scale, and mg or gem scale.

- Measuring spoons and cups: we recommend metal ones as dishwashers and stoves can easily melt plastic ones. I also keep a full set of spoons down to the drop and other micro measurements.

- Airtight glass jars: to keep your extracts from getting too dry.

- Silicone molds: these will be in all shapes and sizes it really depends on the chef what the preferred sizes and shapes are.

- Heat sealer and bags: silver ones like you see most edibles in are available online. This usually counts as childproof containers as well since most bags require scissors and an answered prayer to get open. You can usually get a deal on the sealer online through auctions on used ones and floor models. Try big box stores for decent vacuum sealers locally. Several dispensary supply websites offer great deals on all sizes and the sealer.

- Bottles, jars, and droppers: When making liquid extracts you need to have containers like Kerr jars to hold the big batch, and smaller containers for sales as well. Dropper tops are quite common and all of these are available online in a range of sizes.

- Gloves: a necessity in the food service world, should not be forgotten in this industry for any aspect. Get the ones that fit well for you and last a while. You'll get a chance to test them. We all use a huge amount of them, I go through a box every month.

- Coffee Grinder - The cheap $10 ones that you can get anywhere. I've found having three of them is semi-important and keep each one marked for specific uses. One for coffee, one for spices, and one for your herb. This is far better than any hand grinder you are going to find. This only takes a few pulses to powder most herb, and they don't get clogged up by resin.

Most any other cooking utensil is easily found for the rest of the job. You may want to consider buying a bakers rack if you plan on doing many simultaneous products. This will free up counter space, but will require using the matching baking sheets that will also require purchase. These are all available through Costco, and can be found online for reasonable prices. Some assembly required.

Finally, a chef is only as good as their knives. Make sure you invest in a set you'll find comfortable and easy to sharpen. They come in basic chef kits and I have a used set that are amazing.

Take good care of your tools, as they will be making you money and expanding your horizons. The investment you make into them, will pay off exponentially over time if treated well.

Books

I've already mentioned Ganja Kitchen Revolution in an earlier section about dosing, but there are a few more books I consider must haves for any cannabis chef. I hope these help you as much as they helped me to get where I am now. Green Candy Press is a great source of information altogether. I find many of their books to be spot on for the information I am searching for.

- *The art and science of cooking with cannabis* by Adam Gottlieb

- *Aunt Sandy's Medical Marijuana Cookbook* by Sandy Moriarty

- *Ganja Kitchen Revolution* by Jessica Catalano

- *The Marijuana Cookbook* by S. T. Oner

These four books will be your main textbooks when it comes to learning about cannabis cuisine. They provide an amazing look at dosing, advanced and ancient recipes, and even some great ways to make base ingredients like vanilla and peanut butter.

As for other reading material, I suggest finding any Alton Brown cookbook. He is a great writer and explains food science very well. I have a DVR full of his shows on the Food Network. After all this you know that it's really a matter of ingredient substitution and a little flavor masking. The talent really lies in the already existing culinary talents you possess. Don't forget to raid your grandparents or parents cookbook library. Many old school cookbooks are ingredient based, as compared to modern cookbooks that require more processed ingredients. When you deal with these old recipes you'll find far more ways to infuse cannabis into it while keeping it healthy.

Media

Television cooking shows can also be helpful in the effort to increase culinary aptitude. I've come up with quite a few edibles after seeing a recipe flash across on a competition cooking show. I ended up doing an infused deep fried turkey long before it was cool. I even learned ways of making cupcakes and cookies I hadn't ever considered.

There are also many videos and channels dedicated to food on YouTube and other video sites. These can be great to come up with new ideas, learn techniques, review tools, and discover ingredients. Many are even dedicated to making cannabis cuisine and at a high culinary level. Also videos are a great resource for getting reviews on mass produced edibles you can't get to, or are too far away from and may never try.

Some master edibles chefs have even taken the time to give you industry secrets that just get looked over like a home chef ding a video. Bliss Edibles Master Chef Mrs. Bliss has a great video on how to make the best tinctures. She is also the one who gave me most of the chocolate tips. That company is a great model for aspiring edibles makers. As the company truly cares about their products and the patients that get them. If you are in California, or are planning to visit. Get their stuff, and thank me later. You'll never see edibles the same way again.

You can also find ways to combine base ingredients and tinctures into other carriers. I've even seen a video that explained pairing cannabis, edibles, and wines. There are videos for any topic. If there isn't one. YOU SHOULD MAKE ONE!

Social Media

As the world moves into the cloud. We find ourselves in an amazing new place. With social networks providing people of like minds a place to share their ideas. Expanding their world without ever leaving their living room. We also find many online forums and cannabis specific social apps like High There. Letting cannabis enthusiasts spread there message and help build their brand.

We are no stranger to this. @WonkyEdiblesNV is our twitter handle, and we have a Facebook page as well. You can see us from the minute after tossing around the idea, to making the test foods. This also gives us a chance to share the amazing news that comes out about cannabis on an almost daily basis. This can be a huge help. It can also be a huge pain in the ass. Many states law enforcement are using the web to target some cannabis enthusiasts and businesses. It's really up to you and your comfort level. I have several friends who think we are nuts for sharing this stuff on the internet. I also have some who think that freedom of expression and speech are in my favor. I have made sure to not violate any laws, and am not stupid enough to think I could sell edibles illegally online. The police will catch you if you try. Don't doubt that one bit.

You will find great tips and tricks from people who are sometimes experts in their fields. I've built friendships with manufacturers of lights, seed banks, growers, writers, edible chefs, patients, and even some legends of cannabis. All thanks to social media. So before you say you'd never use social media, don't forget that your edibles may be the next big trend.

Final Thoughts

*"**The dream is free, the hustle is sold separately**"*

- Steve Harvey

I've dreamed of having my own cannabis industry job since 2005. A couple years after medical cannabis was legalized in Nevada. It's now 11 years later. And I ended up a patient who has more knowledge of the inside of the industry than most patients will ever learn.

Dreams are a big thing in the industry. Without the dreamers, we never have the courage to take the industry to new and unique places. Transdermal THC is one of the most unique dreams I've seen yet. Something that should have been an easy idea, took over 15 years to become available in Colorado.

With these dreams, you are only going to go so far. I know firsthand that if you want to get anywhere. You are gonna need to work it. I am not lying, you are going to have to hustle your ass off to get this all going. Don't get dissuaded by naysayers and those who think this is insane. This can be something great, as long as you work for it. You are going to be hitting the pavement, and shaking many hands. Leaving many business cards with many, many people. It may take a while, but if you keep at it. I think you'll find the results promising, if not spectacular.

Treating Addiction With Cannabis

As I finish the book I want to explain my own personal experience treating addiction with cannabis. Something that would make most addiction specialists and doctors cringe.

I had a huge problem in my 20's with amphetamines and other stimulants. I say that broadly, because it was broad. Anything that would work for the pain, and make me feel better. As time in the addiction dragged on. I found myself trying to find a way out.

After finding information on opium addicts being treated. I attempted my own trial.

I bought a quarter pound of cheap pot. I began trying a regimen of smoking until sleep occurred. I knew the first week is always the worst. Withdraw symptoms began and were staved off by the saturation of THC. After a week of this I began modifying the dose to any time I craved the drug, and any time I woke up from the detox period to eat.

Two weeks after I began dropping the dose to the equivalent of 200 mg 6 times a day. A little over a grain of rice of concentrate or FECO oil. About 12 joints for the people unable to get concentrates. Then dropping it over the next month to managed use and as needed. After 3 months I had no interest in the drugs. Total cost was about was $480 of cannabis and the cost of the pipe and butter for the later weeks of edibles use.

You simply need to knock yourself out for that first week and truly saturate your body with THC. Then bring it down slowly and put the dosage where your body loses that craving. I have a few other historical cases to point to, but activist Marc Emery can provide many more recent cases according to Cannabis Culture. He has been helping addicts in Vancouver for years.

I am not an addiction treatment professional, and they will refute this. It's very odd that they'd rather you spend thousands of dollars on inpatient treatment. When you can do this at home with minor supervision for the minor initial detox period. Simply to check on your condition, as any withdraw can be deadly. The nausea will usually subside as the THC level increases in your body. Since cannabis is used to treat epileptics, the chances of withdraw seizures are also reduced. You sleep it all off if you're doing it right. Best wishes for your recovery.

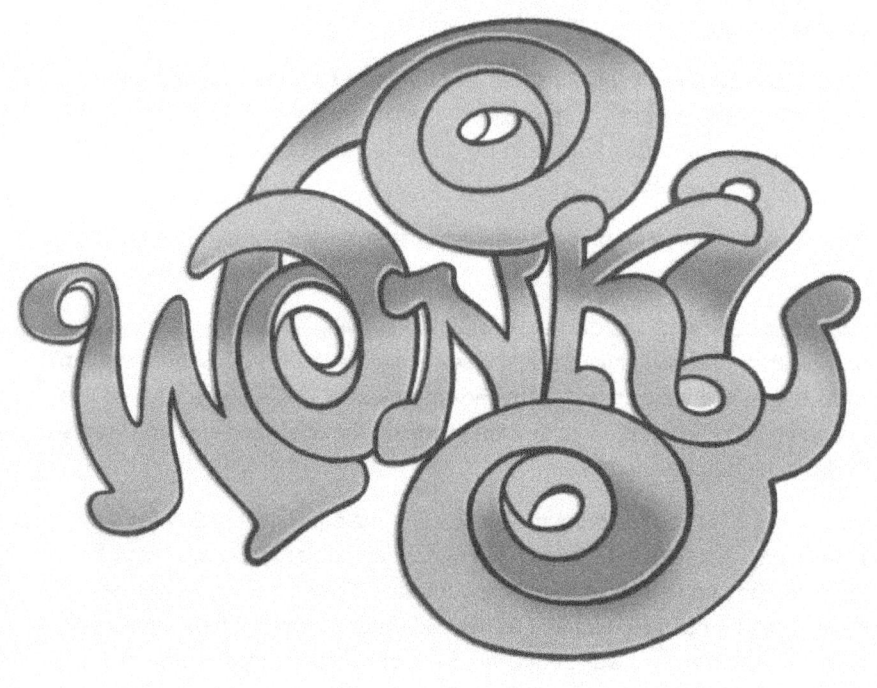

VOLUME 2 COMING SOON